Your own Counter-Current Swimming Pool

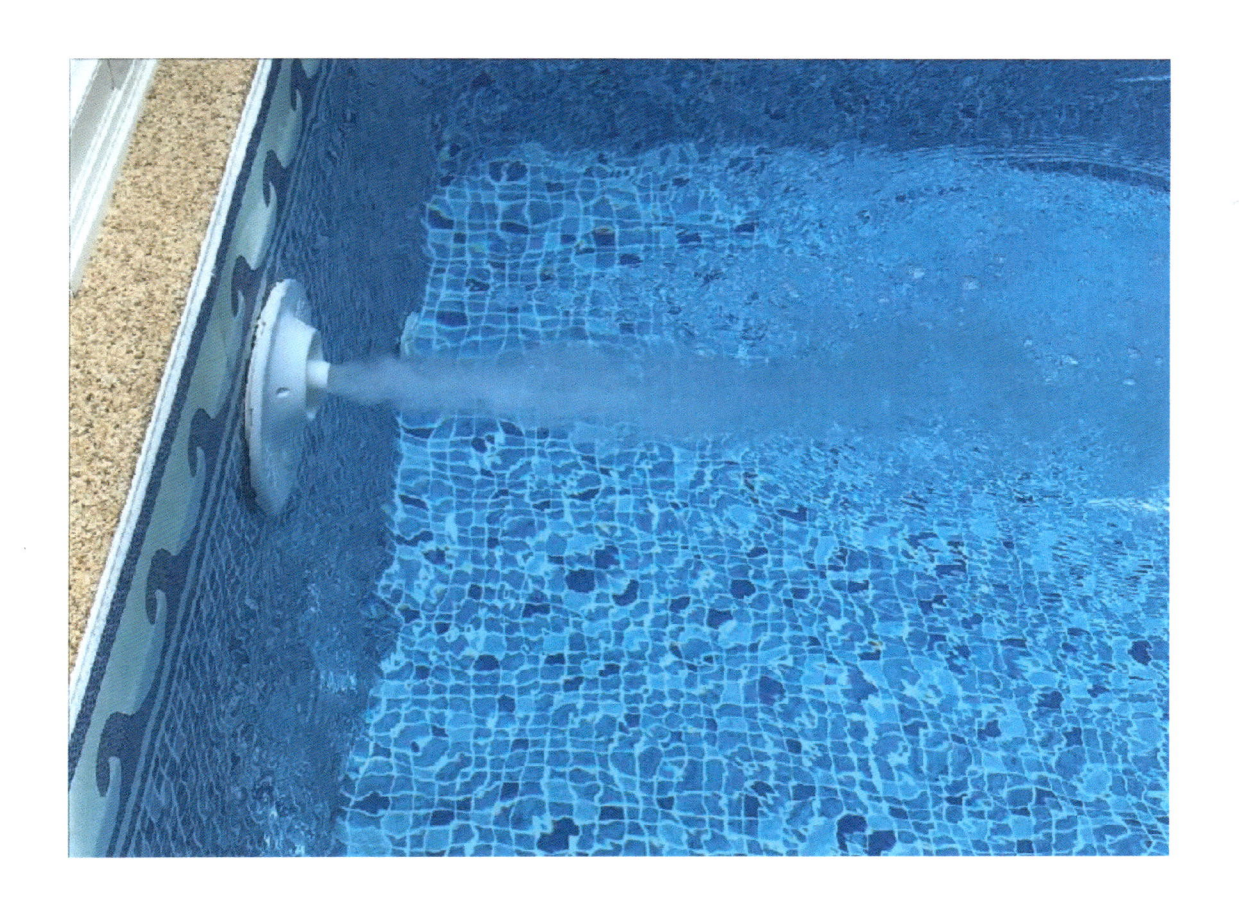

Introduction

You like swimming because it keeps you fit, but sea-swimming is cold, as well as difficult most of the time – and trudging down to the local public pool just spoils your day. So, why not build and operate your own?

This book describes the construction of a swimming pool as well as the operation of its equipment and the management of its water quality. For those who only want a fresh and informative view on managing the pool chemical balance then the second half may be read on its own.

This is a real in-ground pool built for the maintenance of stamina and cardio-vascular fitness by swimming against a variable jet of water. In thirty minutes you can swim a mile - with no turns. Whilst a specific size of pool is used in the text, it is simple to scale-up to the size of pool you require. This design is for an internal or external pool depending on your climate. The equipment and materials are from well-known manufacturers.

There are many "How to" guides on the Internet, covering all the various aspects of swimming pools, and there are many available from equipment and chemical suppliers. This book is for those who want to be involved in the construction of a pool and, in particular want to understand the practical chemistry of their pool as well as how to maintain it.

Table of Contents

The Pool Equipment – layout, operation and management 5

    Introduction 5

    Outline of the Pool's Design and Construction 6

    The Pipework..8

    Drainage 11

The Main Equipment...11

    The Main Pump and Filter 11

    The Heater...12

    UV-Copper Ionizer 14

    The JetVag Counter-Current Pump 15

    Mains water supply 15

    Switching On...15

    Electric Power Supply 16

    The Estimated Cost of Electricity to Operate the Pool 17

    Dehumidifier 18

    Digital Meters to Measure Water Quality 18

    Colorimeters to Measure Water Quality 20

    Constructing the Pool 21

Managing the Quality of the Pool Water...23

Removing visible contaminants..23

    Clear and Odourless Water 23

    Filter the big stuff out 23

    Vacuum the pool floor and walls..24

    Emptying the pool 25

    Adding water 25

Algae 25

Removing invisible contaminants and Sanitising the Pool 26

Clean the People 26

Balancing the Pool Chemistry 26

The pH of the Water 26

Chlorine 27

Enzymes 30

Practical Pool Management or "So, where is all the chlorine going?" 30

Algaecides, Nitrates and Phosphates 32

Cyanuric Acid (CYA) 32

The UV-C Ioniser 32

Hardness and Total Alkalinity 34

Langelier Saturation Index (LSI) – The Practice 35

Total Dissolved Solids (TDS) 35

Balancing the Pool Chemistry – Measurements 36

The pH of the Water 36

Temperature 36

ORP 36

Chlorine 36

Nitrates and Phosphates 36

Hardness 36

Total Alkalinity 36

LSI 37

Copper 37

Total Dissolved Solids (TDS) 37

Balancing the Pool Chemistry – Applying chemicals 37

The Addition of Enzymes and the Removal of Phosphates 38

Maintaining the Free Chlorine and Total Chlorine Levels 38

Hardness and Total Alkalinity 38

Copper 38

Total Dissolved Solids (TDS) 38

Microbe Testing 39

The Chemicals Used 39

Maintenance Sequence *39*

Appendices *40*

Appendix 1: Physical Chemistry 40

Appendix 2: The Theory of The Langelier Saturation Index (LSI) 41

Appendix 3: Hints and tips on joining pipework. 43

Appendix 4: Idealised testing regime 44

Appendix 5: Spreadsheet for monitoring the pool chemistry 45

Appendix 6: Indicative Prices and Costs in £s. 46

Appendix 7: Some Useful References and sources of Interesting Articles. 48

The Pool Equipment – layout, operation and management

Introduction

This chapter is sub-divided into several sub-sections and describes the actual pool structure, the pipe work through which the water moves around the system, the equipment to pump that water and to maintain its quality and finally the outline details of the building work. Each section is deliberately detailed to ensure that you know all the information you need to gather and to understand. Just jump in and wade through it all for now.

The equipment described is off-the-shelf pool equipment and substitutes will be very similar in operation. These may be obtained from any pool equipment supplier. Likewise, the chemicals required can be purchased from any pool chemical supplier and details of those required are given in the Chemicals Used section later. You may need to work with a builder to dig holes, lay concrete and add brickwork. Estimates of the costs involved and the prices of equipment are given in the appendix.

The appendices contain; a spreadsheet to monitor pool chemistry, an idealised testing regime, construction and operating costs, as well as some information on physical chemistry for the curious. The photographs show various details of the actual pool.

If you have ever put two pipes together, or mixed a solution, then you only have to get used to the terminology. There is nothing complicated here - although pool water chemistry is often considered to be very complicated!

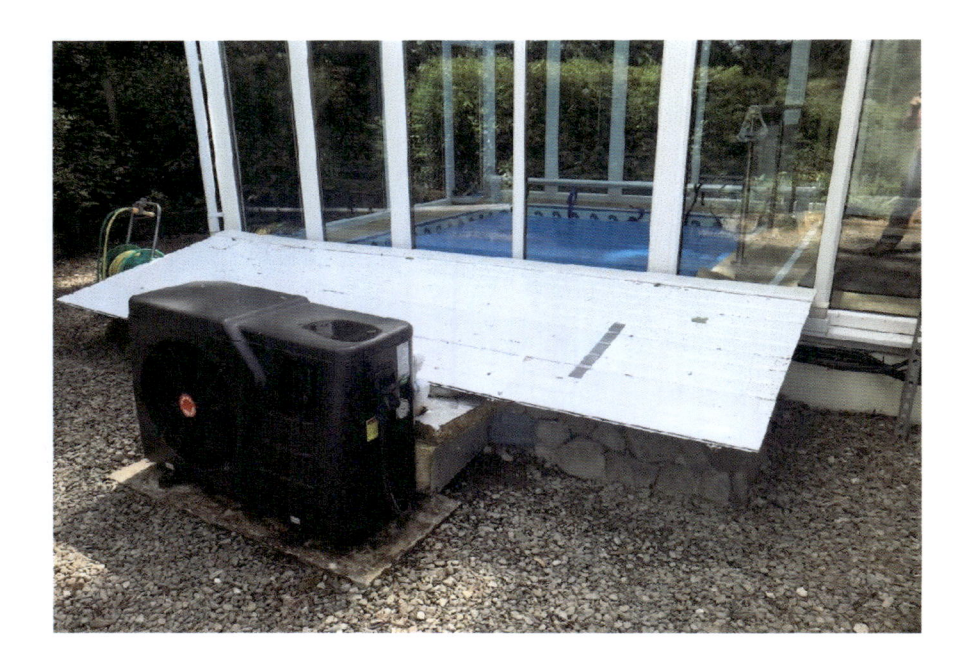

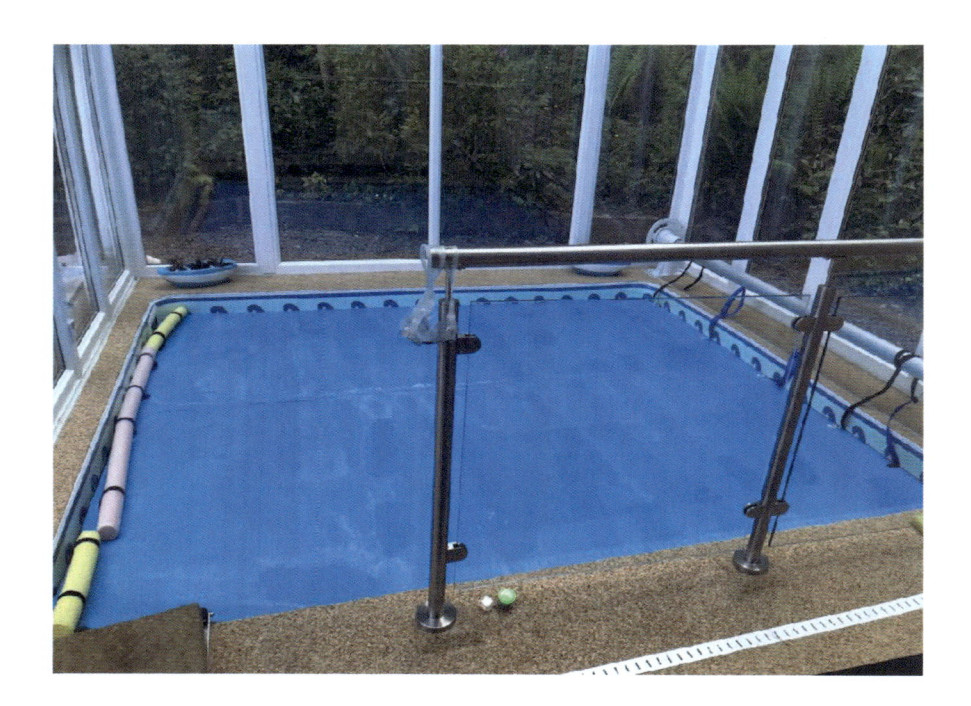

Outline of the Pool's Design and Construction

The pool has a reinforced concrete base set on to a 100 mm thick XPool thermal insulation bed with reinforced block walls also insulated with XPool on the outside. The Xpool forms a complete insulation box around the outside of the concrete and blockwork. Under the Xpool is a layer of sand blinding as shown in the diagram. An off-the-shelf butyl pond liner, sitting on a further sand blinding layer, wraps all of the Xpool and concrete walling, to stop water circulating into and through the Xpool (which would increase the rate of heat loss).

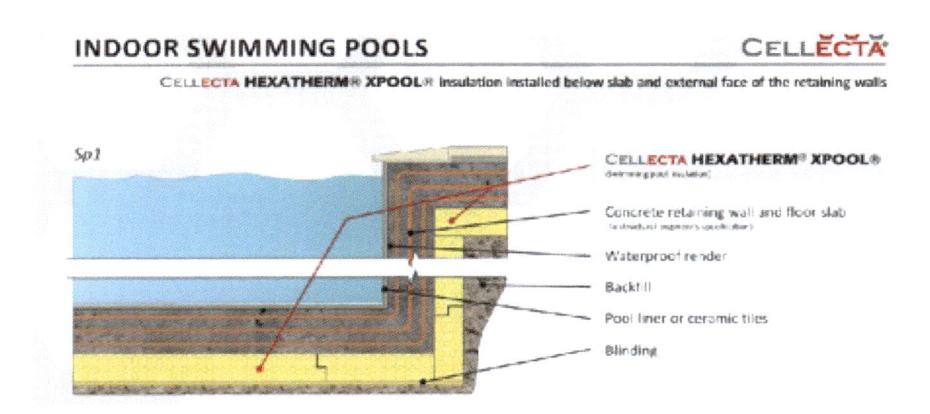

Underfelt and foam padding covers the pool bottom, with underfelt on the walls, beneath the pool liner. The liner was produced to fit the actual dimensions of the pool in mm (note that it is not exactly square):

2615 By 2625
3015 By 3005
1385 By 1385 (Depth)

The pool liner is fitted into the pool liner-lock at the rim of the pool and held in place by a trim. The pool surround is SureSet, consisting of crushed marble (3 mm) embedded in resin. This sits on a cement screed over the pool block-work and the concrete entrance-floor, under which is further insulation.

The water output ports (i.e. from the pool) are near the floor of the pool on the same wall as the counter current port and the skimmer. The input ports are on the opposite wall near the top. The vacuum port is on the same side as the pool light. These ports and the counter-flow and the skimmer flanges are fitted so that they sandwich the pool's liner between two seals (like 'O' rings). The components of each flange are held together with screws. Since these screws are into plastic it is important that they are not over-tightened as the thread in a flange can be easily stripped. Note that there are usually several unused screw holes.

The structure of the pool gives a size of 1.5 metres deep, 3 metres long, 2.6 metres wide. This means a potential volume of 11700 litres. The pool water height, to the middle of the skimmer's mouth, is about 1.3 metres giving a volume of water of 10,000 litres.

When the pool is not in use a cover (on the roller) should always be in place to reduce evaporation. For long periods is a set of Cellotex blocks, shrink wrapped in plastic can be used for greater insulation. These can fit together and be positioned on top of the cover to retain as much heat as possible.

The Pipework

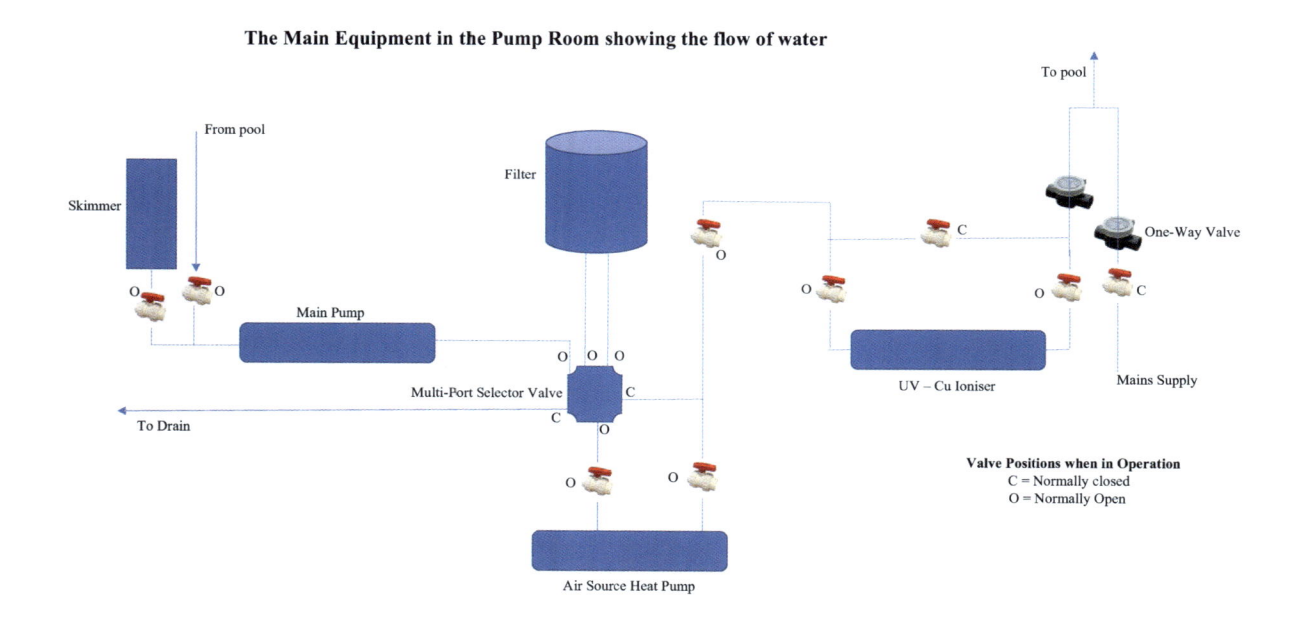

The Main Equipment in the Pump Room showing the flow of water

Valve Positions when in Operation
C = Normally closed
O = Normally Open

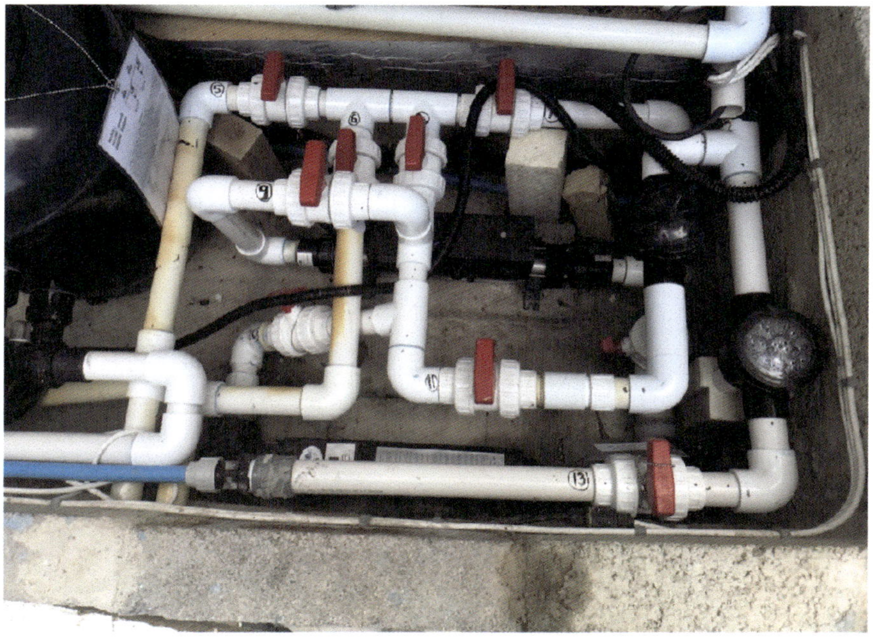

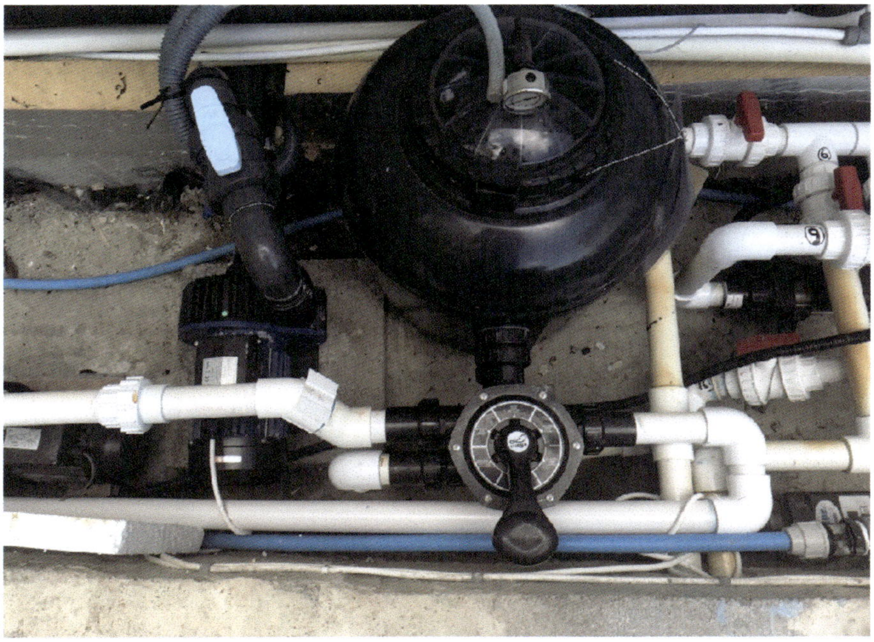

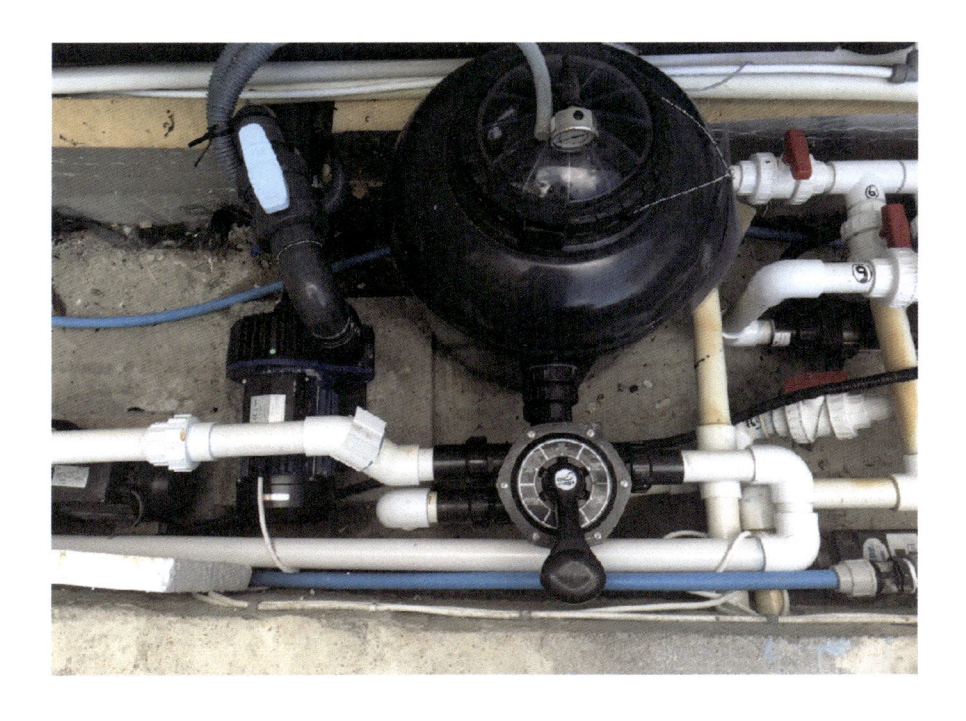

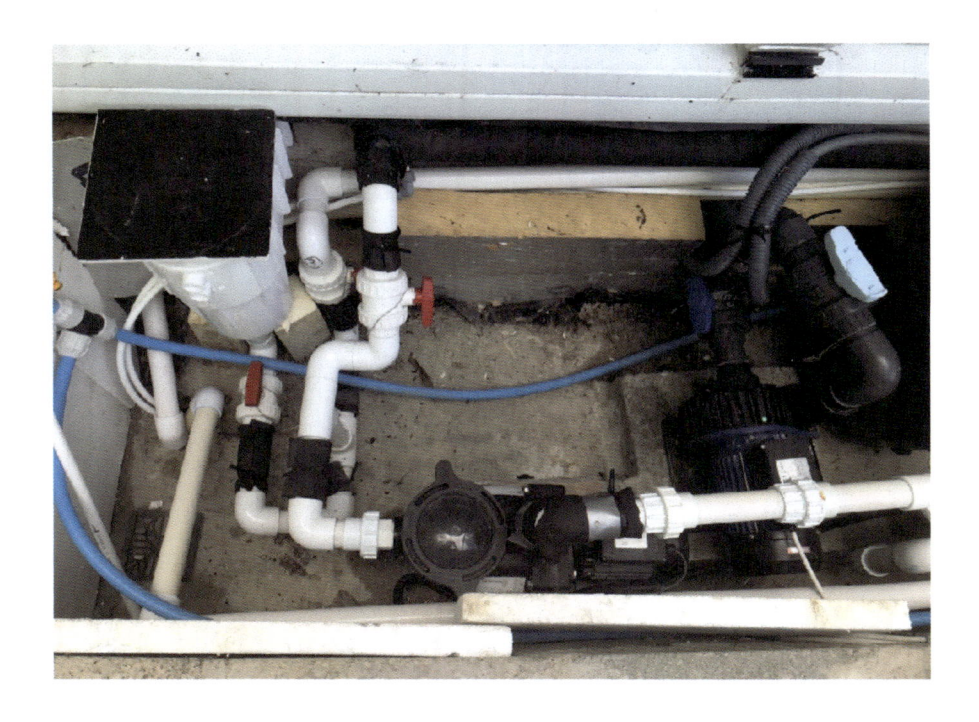

The pipework is Certikin 1.5 inch (internal diameter) Class 'C' thick-walled white pipe. Black insulation sleeves are used to retain heat but these are not entirely necessary as the thick pipe walls do not even get warm. The external diameter of the pipe is 2 inches. Pipe joints are sealed with PVC cement (blue, WDF-05 Griffin). In the appendix is a section of hints and tips on joining pipes.

There are also joints with 'O' ring seals (particularly the valves) and some with screw threads sealed with PTFE tape. All joints need to be monitored for leaks. The diagram shows the pipework detail.

The vacuum point and the inlet and outlet ports are standard Certikin. The 12 Volt SeaMaid LED pool light is fitted onto a modified Certikin joint with its armoured cable passing under the floor to the transformer and the mains.

The Jet-Vag counter-current pump is on a separate water loop to the main system, using 2 inch grey pipes. It takes water directly out of the pool and pushes it back in, mixed with air.

The mains water inlet is connected directly to the pool input pipe through a non-return valve. A further non-return valve prevents water flowing backwards towards the pump.

There are numerous valves within the pipework with 'O' rings that are greased with silicone (and they should be silicone greased again after being disturbed). The main pieces of equipment (the UV-C ioniser, the air-source heat pump (primary heater) and the 9kW electric heater (a secondary heater that is not required in practice)) each have three valves to enable them to be bypassed and isolated and, if necessary, removed. In addition the vacuum-cleaner line, the pool outlet lines and the skimmer line have individual valves.

These valves allow you to:

1. Adjust the balance of flows down the various pipes, i.e. to lower the flow rate through a unit by partially closing off a valve (although this has not proved necessary).
2. Isolate and remove units (e.g. the UV-C ioniser) for maintenance and allow the flow to by-pass that unit.
3. Fully open or close pipework during normal operation.

Note that the ball inside a valve will come out if the valve's screw clamp is removed whilst there is pressure behind it.

There are 15 valves in the system and under normal operation their positions are shown in the following table.

Valve No.	Unit Name	Normal Status	Description
1	Skimmer	Open	Output from skimmer
2	Drains	Open	Output from pool drains
3	Vacuum	Closed	Output from vacuum cleaner point
4	ASHP - In	Open	Inlet to air-source heat pump (primary heater)

5	ASHP Bypass	Closed	Bypass to air-source heat pump
6	ASHP - Out	Open	Outlet from air-source heat pump
7	EH - In	Closed	Inlet to electric heater (secondary heater)
8	EH Bypass	Open	Bypass to electric heater (secondary heater)
9	EH – Out	Closed	Outlet from electric heater (secondary heater)
10	UV – In	Open	Inlet to UV / Ioniser
11	UV Bypass	Closed	Bypass to UV / Ioniser
12	UV – Out	Open	Outlet from UV / Ioniser
13	Mains – In	Closed	Mains water inlet to the system
14	CC – In	Open	Inlet to counter current pump
15	CC – Out	Open	Outlet from counter current pump

Drainage

The main drainage line is from the filter to the drain and is used mainly for the backwashing cycle. There is also a line to this drain from the main drainage channel of the pool room, as well as small-bore pipework that connects the drainage channels at the sides of the pool. These channels are imbedded in the SureSet resin flooring.

This pool uses a catchment tank connected to the drain. This avoids large flows of water running down the hill on this site and causing landslip but will also act as a buffer between the pool and the main drains. The tank can take roughly a foot of the pool water (2000 Lt) before it must be drained itself.

The pool can be fully drained through the Mega filter pipework or, alternatively, submersible electric water-pumps are available that can be dropped to the bottom of the pool for rapid emptying.

The Main Equipment

The details given here are the main points for operating the pool, recognising that the manuals provided are both brief and often in poor English.

The Main Pump and Filter

The Pentair SuperFlo Pump (3/4 HP, i.e. 0.6 kW) sucks water from the bottom of the pool through the two drain ports, as well as from the skimmer. It is either on or off. The actual flow rate in the system depends upon the restrictions caused by the pipework and the equipment along the line, but this pump has a nominal value of 15,000 Litres per hour i.e. 4 litres per second, with a 10 metre head.

It is possible to connect the pump so that it is controlled by the Air-Source Heat Pump (ASHP) – and electricians will automatically connect the system this way – but this prevents independent operation to enable, for example, back-washing the filter. It is better that the pump operates independently. Note that when the water flow is well established it is not apparent through the sight glass that there is water in the pump. BE CAREFUL that the pump is not operating without appropriate valves being open or without water halfway up the skimmer to avoid the pump sucking air. Otherwise the pump may overheat and be damaged.

The pump pushes all the water into the Mega SMG500 filter via the filter control valve. Under normal operation this is set to 'filter' which channels the water through the sand within the body of the filter tank to remove debris. The sand is 100 kg of Grade 1 Hydro-Pro, Eco-Pure glass media of 0.5 to 1.0 mm size. When the pool was first operated the pressure gauge at the top of the filter read 85 psi. The pressure will rise as the sand becomes dirty but should return to this value after it is cleaned by backwashing. Other settings on the filter valve redirect the water when, for example, bypassing it or backwashing.

The Heater

This is a Hydro-Pro + Premium 10 air-source heat pump (ASHP). It is operational all year round, requiring little maintenance. It has a cooling as well as a heating mode and there is also an automatic mode with an internal timer.

There is a single controller interface showing the various modes and settings for temperature, time, etc. The manual is not clear about the setting procedure, so this is how to programme it.

1. Turn on the main pump since the heater will not work unless the pump is driving water through it.
2. Press the on/off button on the integral display to switch the heater on. The large number is the current water inlet temperature and the small number is the outlet temperature. Although this 'on/off' button starts the heater there will be a delay as the heater resets itself.
3. The time button allows you to set the time and set a timing sequence for the automatic mode. Neither is required since the timer in the fuse box provides control under Economy 10. Make sure that there are no 'on' or 'off' symbols next to the time display as this indicates that a timing setting may have been made and the heater will then not work outside of those set times.
4. The Mode/Set button allows you to select the mode. Pressing it cycles through 'cooling', 'heating' and 'automatic' symbols. Leave it on the 'heating' setting.
5. The up and down arrows allow you to adjust the value of the Target Temperature. Press one of them to start setting the target temperature. When doing so, the Inlet Temperature reading becomes the Target Temperature reading and flashes. When the Target Temperature required has been set, <u>press the Mode/Set button to fix it in</u>. If you don't then the Target will revert to the original setting. Similarly, if you press the on/off button whilst you are resetting the Target any changes will be cancelled and it will revert to the original setting.
6. The ASHP will drive the outlet temperature of the water until the inlet temperature reaches the target temperature.

The ratio of heating provided to work required is called the Coefficient of Performance (COP – see graph). Higher COPs equate to lower operating costs. This heat pump has a Coefficient of Performance of 4.5 at an air temperature of 20°C falling to 2.5 at 0°C, maintaining the water at 27°C, but draws only 1.7kW (c.f. a typical pool electric heater drawing 9kW).

Particularly during the winter, operating the ASHP during the daytime (assuming you are using off-peak electricity – Economy 10 in the UK – between 13:00 and 16:00 GMT) will mean heating during the maximum COP available. The air temperature will fall closer to freezing at night lowering the available COP. The high degree of insulation around the pool enables the pool's temperature to hold steady even during the night. Nevertheless after backwashing and part-filling with cold water it will take longer for the pool to get back to temperature in the winter because of the lower COP.

This Air-Source Heat Pump is designed for pools of up to 40,000 litres (four times this pool's volume) and, since the purchase and running costs of heat pumps of various sizes are about the same, this allows for a more rapid heating of the pool water for little extra expense. The required flow rate through the heater is approximately 0.8 litres per second (i.e. 3000 litres per hour).

The term 'R407C' refers to the refrigerant gas (or rather mixture of gases) that is used in the ASHP. It is currently the most environmentally-friendly hydrofluorocarbon available.

Note that a secondary heater can be seen in some of the pictures. Whilst this remains in the circuit it has been totally superseded by the ASHP. This is a 9kW electric heater.

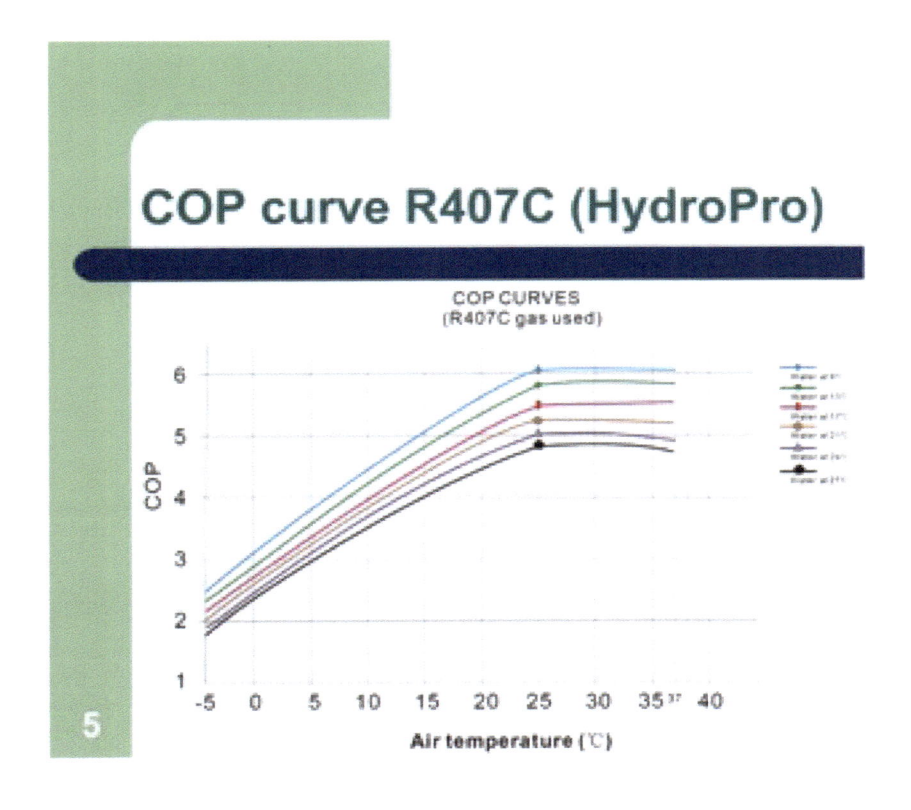

COP curve R407C (HydroPro)

UV-Copper Ionizer

This is a 75W Blue Lagoon UV-C Ioniser that kills organisms (i.e. bacteria, virus or algae) by exposing their DNA to UV radiation (causing damage by a reaction between two molecules of thymine in the nucleic acid) or by ionising them with copper ions. The UV lamp radiates at 253nm at peak. This is above the range of 180–200nm where UV dissociates the chlorine sanitiser (although there will be some reduction) but is within the range of 245–365nm where the dissociation of chloramines (the smelly products of chlorine sanitation) occurs.

The copper ioniser (if activated) releases trace amounts of copper ions into the water that attach to an organism's cell surface proteins eventually killing them. Ionisation, like the UV, purifies water slowly in comparison to chlorine. Initially the ioniser will not be used (copper in the pool can turn hair green).

The water from the heaters flows through the UV-C Ioniser, before flowing back into the pool.

Notes:
1. The stainless steel of the UV-C will corrode if salt is introduced into the water.
2. The device is mounted so that there is always water in the UV-C and there are ball valves to allow isolation and removal as well as for flow control.
3. When plugged in, the UV-C lamp starts automatically and requires no adjustment. It does not switch off if there is no flow of water.
4. The UV-C lamp may need replacement every year and is positioned to enable isolation and extraction.
5. The amount of UV radiation (as a percentage of the total radiation emitted by the lamp) can be as low as 10%. The actual energy dose (assuming 75 watts over a tube area of 75cm and 10% efficiency) is about 100mJ (0.1 Watt/sq.cm/sec). At this dosage, and with a wide spectrum, the radiation should both kill bacteria and break up chloramine contaminants.
6. There will be a certain level of copper in ordinary water and the total level of copper should not exceed 0.7ppm to avoid copper deposits and discolouration.

7. The ioniser automatically switches off after 14 days of operation to ensure that the copper concentration is measured and adjusted to be within tolerance.
8. The copper rods will need cleaning using a copper brush and eventually a proprietary cleaner as well – probably once a year.

Before using the ioniser, the pH of the pool must be at the correct level of 7.4 otherwise the copper ions will precipitate out onto surfaces, showing as a greenish deposit – particularly at the skimmer. Having measured the initial copper ion concentration of the pool, the ioniser can be switched on and adjusted to maintain a level of between 0.4 and 0.7ppm, target 0.5ppm.

The ioniser's display shows a number between 00 and 99 that represents the status of the copper emissions. If the copper content is low (measured by a strip) then pushing the + button will start the ioniser and increase the emission of copper. Adjust marginally (e.g. to 33) and wait for a week before measuring again. If the copper level is too high move the display to 00 (off) and wait for a week before adjusting the copper emissions. The ioniser can be switched off permanently by setting it to 00.

The JetVag Counter-Current Pump

This pump has a power of 2.3kW and is started and stopped from the pneumatic stop/start button on the faceplate. There is also a remote control that starts and stops the motor by pressing button 'B' (button 'A' has no function). There are two ball valves (14 & 15) that isolate the JetVag from its pump for maintenance. These are normally left fully open. By slightly closing the valves, the flow rate into the pool could be reduced but this is not the best way to manage the flow rate. BE CAREFUL that this pump is not started without both of the valves being open, otherwise it will break!

There are two 20mm blue reinforced pipes coming from the faceplate into the pump room. One of these has a 5mm clear pipe that is the pneumatic control pipe going to the cabinet containing the electrics. Take care to ensure that this is not squashed or trapped to ensure that the pneumatic signal is not cut off. The second blue pipe supplies air to mix with the water pulled out and injected back into the pool. This pipe must be held above the pool level or water will siphon out of the pool.

Inside the pool, within the Jet-Vag faceplate is the output pipe. With the Jet-Vag <u>off</u> this pipe can be moved around to adjust the angle of the flow into the pool. Be careful not to have the water flow shooting out of the pool. Inside the output-pipe are two vanes that overlap. By rotating the pipe (whilst the Jet-Vag is off) these vanes are made to overlap to a greater or lesser extent thus changing the pressure experienced by the swimmer. In addition the angle of the output-pipe can be changed, or the water-jet may be approached from the side, to reduce the pressure experienced.

Mains water supply

The volume of the pool water will decrease by evaporation or after transferring dirty water into the waste line. The water main is connected through its own valve (number 13) with a one-way valve preventing pool water going into the mains and a one-way valve preventing any mains water travelling backwards through the pipework towards the main pump.

It takes about two hours to fill the pool from the bottom of the Jet Vag fascia to the middle of the skimmer mouth. In that time it is very easy to forget that the valve is open and the pool is filling! You need a way to ensure you remember, such as a timer. Do not have the main pump on whilst mains water is being added since this will cause back-pressure onto the non-return valves and competition between water flows.

Switching On

Ensure that all the equipment is (as far as possible) full of water before starting. The pool level should be halfway up the skimmer. Open the appropriate valves (1 and 2) to let water flow into the Pentair pump to the filter and the rest of the equipment. Make sure you have all valves open or closed as appropriate (see 'pipework' section).

If the level of water falls below the skimmer mouth the pump will pull air in through the skimmer line and you'll see bubbles being pumped into the pool. This is not good for the pump and needs to be watched for, as pool water level will slowly fall. Follow the instructions to top up the water level (see prior section).

Electric Power Supply

Main points:
1. The pump and UV are plugged into sockets that are timed and operate during the cheap-rate electricity ('Off Peak', Economy 10 or E10) available in the UK.
2. The pool light is plugged into a socket that is not timed and (like the counter current pump) there is a remote control to operate this light.
3. The ASHP has its own switch but this is also timed and under E10. The ASHP switches off automatically when the pump is not operating.
4. The JetVag counter-current pump is connected to its own controller and from there directly to the fuse box.
5. This fuse box is connected to the rest of house's electricity supply through its own main switch.

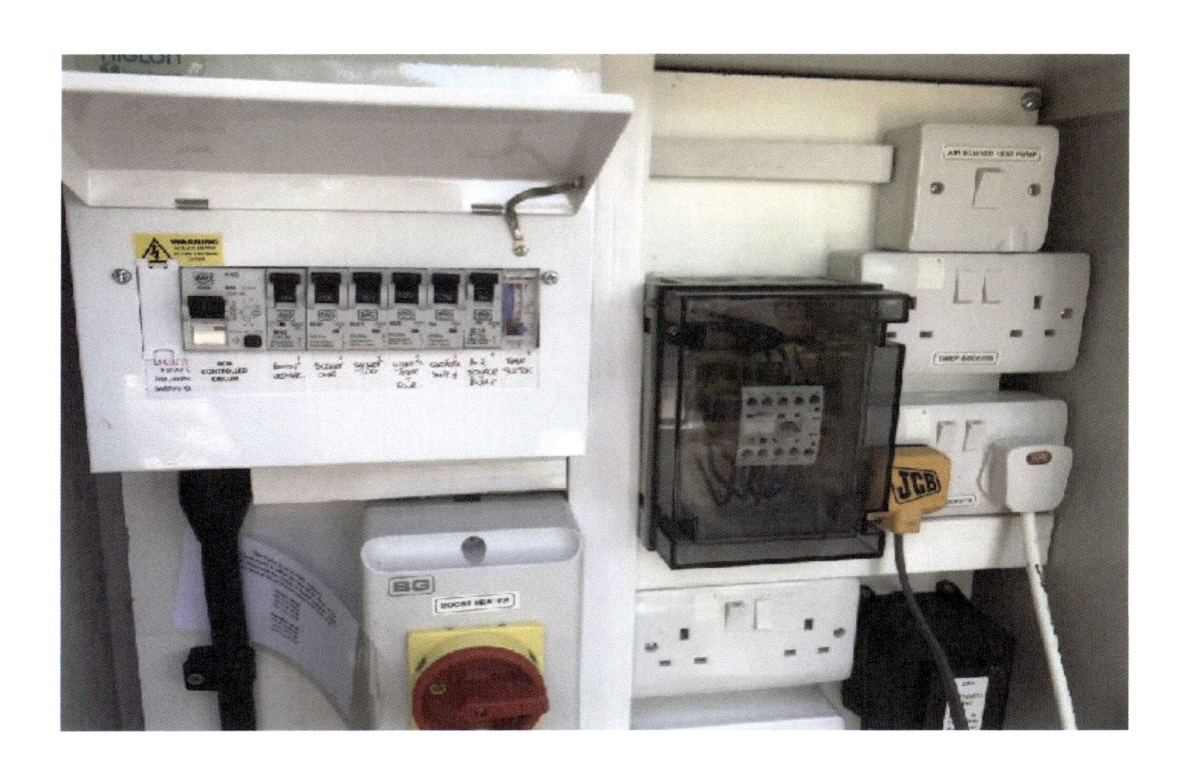

The electricity usage can be divided as follows:
1. The counter-current pump, at 2.3 kW, is likely to be used at prime time (morning and evening). In addition, the lights (LED) and cover roller motor (if fitted) will be used at the same time but their power demand is very low.

2. A small (up to 0.5kW) dehumidifier (discussed later) is operated under the control of an hygrometer. This will usually respond quickly to the pool being used but is set for a low kW usage.
3. The balance of the equipment consists of the main pump (0.6kW), the primary (ASHP) heater (1.7kW) and the UV C-ioniser (75W) that are intended to operate at E10 off-peak times.

Electricity Usage Notes

1. kW is a measure of power. kW Hr (described as 'Units' in the UK) is a measure of energy.
2. The energy that needs to be added to raise a mass of water (10,000 litres = 10,000 kg.) from 10°C to 30°C = the specific heat of water (4.19 kJ/kg.) x 10000 kG x 20 °C / 3600 = 232 kW. Hr. Therefore, the 10 kW heater would take 232/10 = 23 Hrs to heat the volume of water from 10 to 30 degrees. Note that the '3600' term converts seconds to hours since a Watt = Joule /sec
3. The 1.7kW air-source heat pump, with a COP (= heat provided /work done) of say 5, is equivalent to nearly 10 kW (1.7 'X' 5 = 8.5 kW). However, the COP will be lower in winter.
4. The ASHP is operating for only 5 hours per day to maintain the pool temperature at about 30°C. Water quality needs to be monitored as well as temperature since the pump is not operating continuously.
5. The main heating is during the three hours of daylight that off-peak electricity is provided. This is when the COP will be at the highest (since the day-time temperature is higher than the night).

The Estimated Cost of Electricity to Operate the Pool

These are the charges for both on and off peak usage with Economy 10 which provides the opportunity, in the UK, to operate the pool using cheap electricity.

	On Peak	Off Peak
£ per kW/Hr ('Unit')	0.25	0.11

Equipment	Power kW	On-Peak Hrs/day	Off-Peak Hrs/day	kW Hrs /day	£ per day	£ p.a.	£ p.m.	*Off-Peak 5 Hrs/day*	*£ p.m.*	Off-Peak 7 Hrs/day	£ p.m.
C. C. Pump	2.300	0.5		1.15	0.29	105	8.7		*8.7*		8.7
Main Pump	0.600		10	6	0.66	241	20.1	*5*	*10.0*	7	14.1
Dehumidifier	0.600	2		1.2	0.30	110	9.1		*9.1*		9.1
ASHP	1.700		10	17	1.87	683	56.9	*5*	*28.4*	7	39.8
UV/C	0.075		10	0.75	0.08	30	2.5	*5*	*1.3*	7	1.8
Totals				26.1	3.2	1168	**97**		*58*		73

Note that typically a timer in the fuse box is not very accurate so the on/off times have been adjusted to ensure that it does not switch over during peak times. The timer is actually set to GMT (winter), but there is no need to adjust the time of the clock or the on/off times with the switch to British Summer Time because the on/off times change by the same hour.

Winter on/off	Summer on/off
00:15 to 05:00	01:15 to 06:00
13:15 to 16:00	14:15 to 17:00
20:15 to 22:00	21:15 to 23:00

Dehumidifier

Inside the poolroom is a dehumidifier initially set to 70% Relative Humidity (RH). This is intended to operate so that any condensation that appears, primarily on the glass, is quickly removed. The water that is evaporated contains a little chlorine and, although the poolroom is mainly glass and uPVC, maintaining a low humidity should prevent problems such as mould, corrosion or algae growth. It is often recommended for a pool room to be below 60% RH but the condition of the pool room remains good. The dehumidifier has various settings but the maximum power it can draw is about 0.5 kW.

The following graph shows that for a room temperature at 20 °C, the air will hold some 11-12g of water per kilogram of air at 80% RH. The dew point, when water condenses out onto the coldest surfaces, is the matching 100% RH point, which is 16°C. So, anything with a temperature of 16°C or less will suffer condensation.

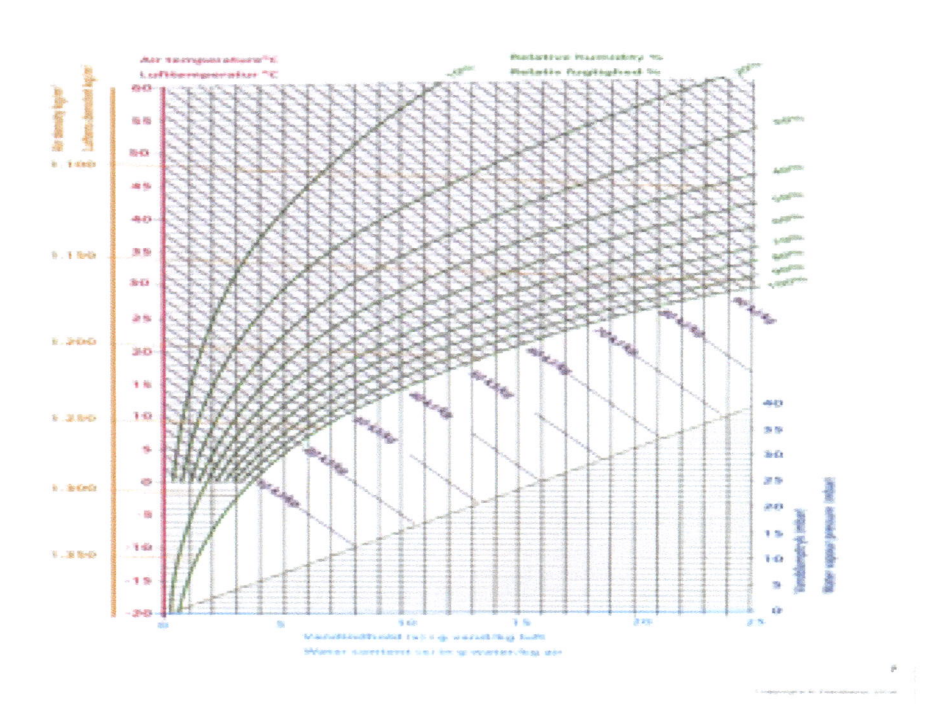

Digital Meters to Measure Water Quality

There are currently three key meters available to measure elements of the water quality, (they are all based on ion conduction in water):

1. Total Dissolved Solids (TDS). This meter actually measures electrical conductivity (EC) but the meter converts this measure to TDS in ppm. Whilst, technically, this is not a very accurate measure it is excellent for determining when the TDS is too high and water needs replacing.
2. pH. This is the most critical meter. It requires calibration with the standard solutions to ensure pH of the pool is maintained accurately to 7.4 +/- 0.2.
3. Redox or Oxidation Reduction Potential (ORP). This measures the potential of any sanitiser in the pool. It is the oxidising potential of the water (oxidative disinfection)

that is important for sanitation, not the level of chlorine. This is an expensive meter (about £250) and there is a calibration solution and storage solution necessary.

The requirement is for rapid disinfection to ensure the protection of bathers. The following graph from Eutech Pty Ltd (see appendix 7) illustrates the E.coli kill time as a function of ORP. For this pool with limited use (and very clean bathers) an ORP of 750 should be excellent.

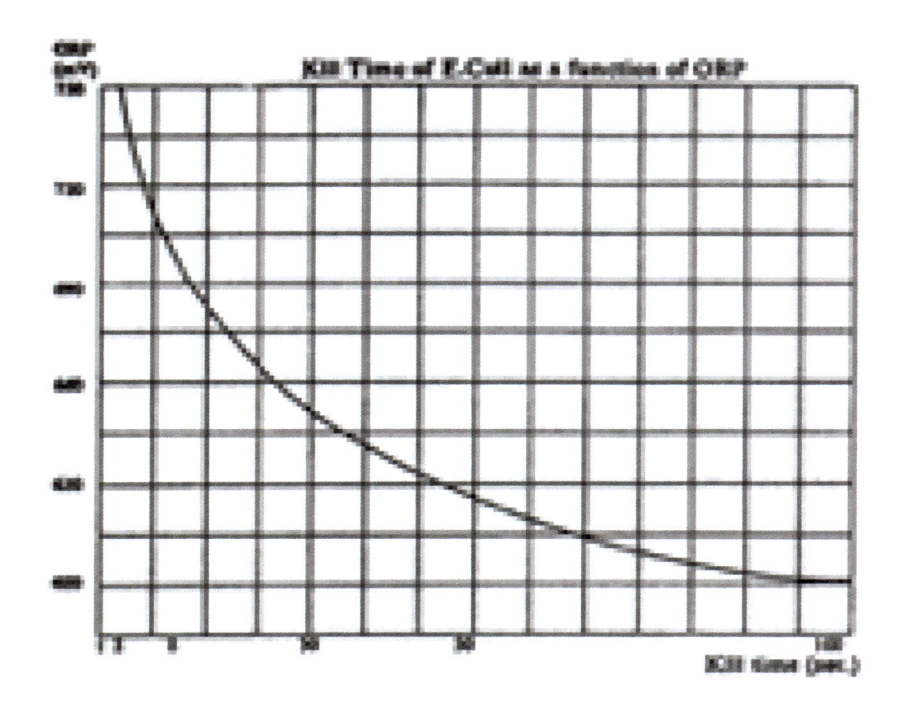

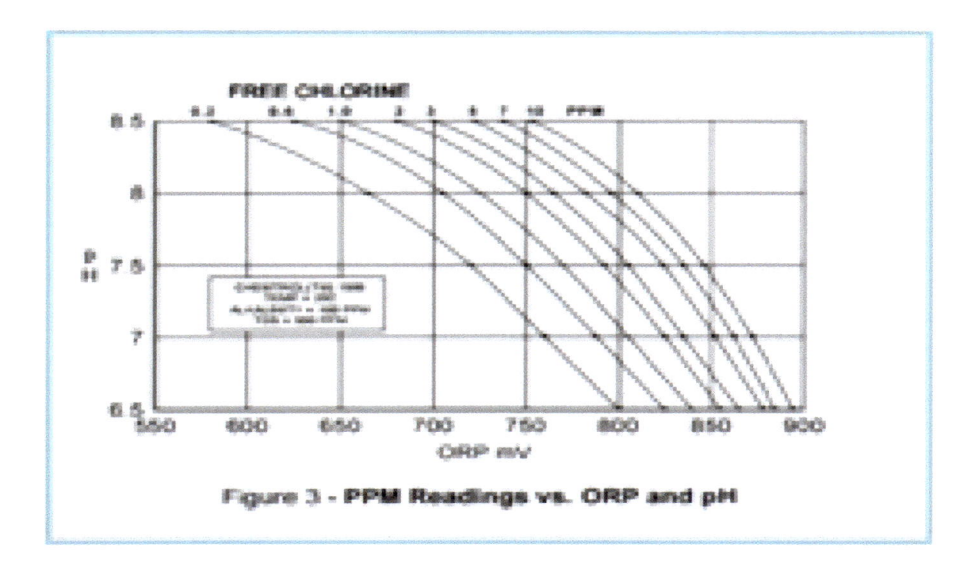

Figure 3 - PPM Readings vs. ORP and pH

The second graph shows the ORP reading for various chlorine ppm at a fixed pH. For this pool, using UV, then, provided TDS is low (<500ppm) and the pH is 7.4, only a small amount of chlorine, about 0.5ppm, *should* be necessary. In this situation if the ORP reads 750mV then the oxidation potential of the added chlorine would be ideal. Note that the inclusion of Cyanuric Acid (CYA) stabiliser into the chlorine can lower the ORP reading significantly.

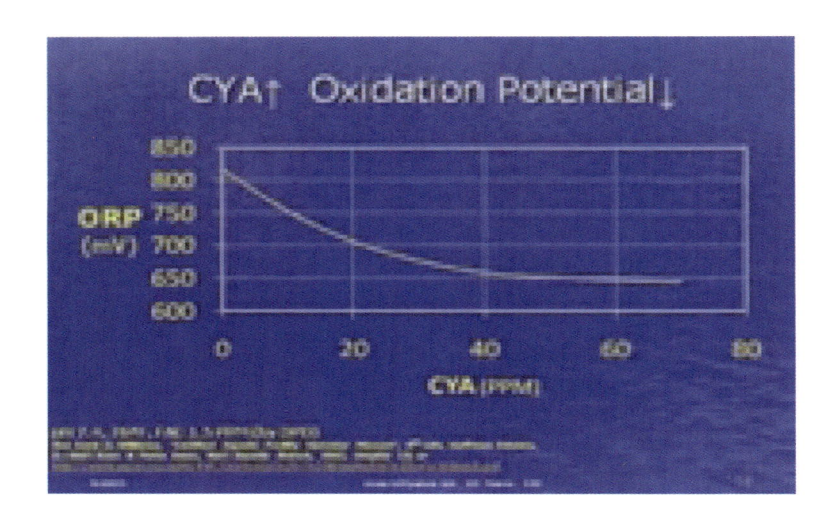

Operationally there is an issue with using ORP measurements (discussed in detail in a paper by Myronl - see appendix 7). It is not uncommon for an ORP sensor to take 10 minutes to arrive at a stable reading and that can make its regular measurement rather tedious - few people will wait. Some form of mount to allow the meter to be held in the flowing water for the ORP to settle is required.

Knowing the ORP and the pH does not tell you the actual free chlorine in the pool but it can be inferred from the above graph and confirmed by measurement. However, digital meters can quickly, and reasonably accurately, tell the status of the pool in terms of temperature, TDS, pH and ORP - ideal for frequent checks. Details of the use of these meters is given in the sections covering the management of water quality. Note that they will require both cleaning and calibration at regular intervals as well as storage in the appropriate solution (see equipment maintenance for details).

Colorimeters to Measure Water Quality

The measurement of chlorine, water hardness and total alkalinity, as well as copper, phosphates and nitrates all use colour as the basis for measuring the ppm in the pool water. Often this is achieved by dipping a stick in the pool water, on which are spots of appropriate chemical, and observing the colour change of the spot against a chart marked in ppm. This is very inaccurate - especially if you have any degree of colour-blindness. The manufacture of the sticks is often poor and the ability to see the appropriate reading is at least 'difficult'. For something so important as the chemical balance of the pool these are not worth the wasted time and inaccurate readings - but they are cheap.

Most pool companies sell multitask stations that are based on adding chemicals to a water sample and observing a colour against a colour chart marked in ppm. Whilst they are used extensively, they fall into the same category - although they are not cheap.

Since these measurements are so important it is far better to use the Hanna products (or those of other lab equipment suppliers) in particular for total and free chlorine, ORP and pH. Companies, such as Seachem, provide Copper, Nitrate and Phosphate tests kits that are intended for aquariums and these provide sufficient accuracy.

There are also titration methods available to accurately measure water hardness and total alkalinity, as well as copper and phosphates. These show a fairly clear colour change that provides sufficiently accurate readings. Details of these are also provided in the appendix.

Equipment Maintenance

The heater, both pumps and the mechanical parts of the filter do not need regular maintenance (see manuals).

The UV lamp should be replaced after a number of hours e.g. every year (around £100). The copper rod can become covered in deposits, so it should be cleaned with a copper wire brush after dipping in a cleaner. The element will eventually be used up.

To maintain the Mega500 filter's efficiency, clean the filter sand every year using a filter-cleansing product (e.g. Blue Horizons' Filter Cleaner).

The pH and ORP metres may need regular calibration (say, every three months) and certainly regular cleaning. Calibration powders and distilled water are available for these from eBay. Hanna Instruments supply calibration standard solutions (e.g. HI 7022 and HI 7021) for the ORP meter and also a pre-treatment solution (HI 7092 for oxidising pre-treatment). Both meters should be stored in an electrode storage solution (e.g. HI 70300L).

Constructing the Pool

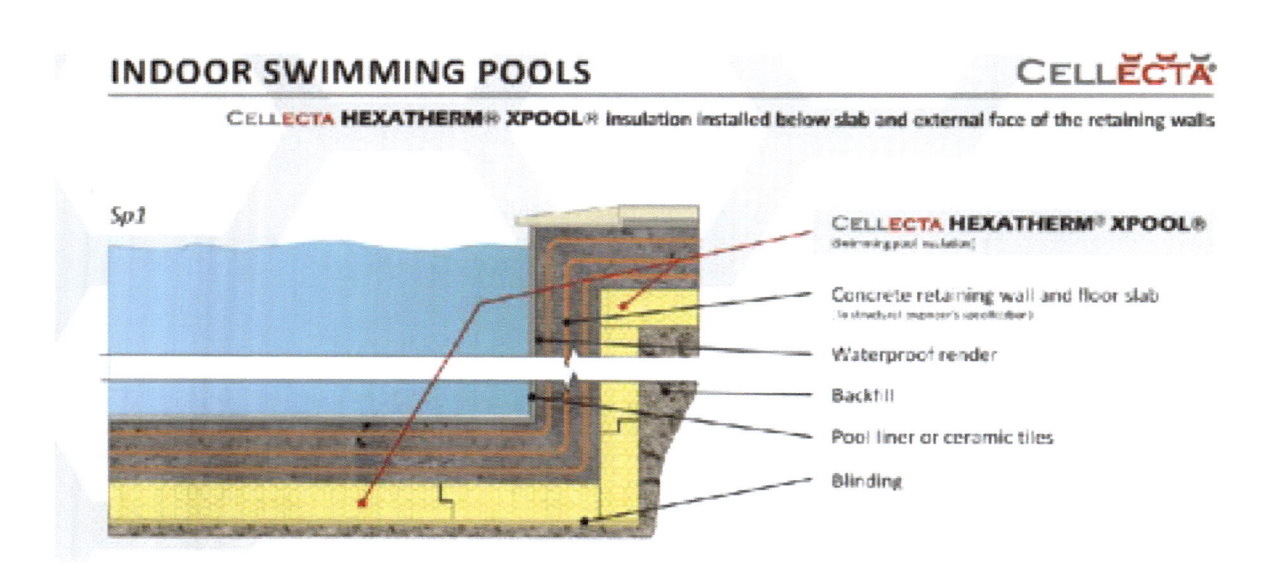

INDOOR SWIMMING POOLS — CELLECTA

CELLECTA HEXATHERM XPOOL insulation installed below slab and external face of the retaining walls

- CELLECTA HEXATHERM XPOOL swimming pool insulation
- Concrete retaining wall and floor slab (to structural engineer's specification)
- Waterproof render
- Backfill
- Pool liner or ceramic tiles
- Blinding

This description is given in the sequence that this pool was constructed.

1. The natural drainage of the area and roof water drains were checked and any improvements required were made. A new drain was installed in the pump room area for the collection for any wastewater from the pool before disposal.

2. A clear area of land 6 metres by 6 metres was taken and using an excavator a square hole 2.5 metres deep and 3.5 metres by 3 metres square. Some 26 cubic metres of soil (50 to 75 barrows) weighing about 40 tonnes was then relocated on the site.

3. About 25 mm of building sand was then laid on the bottom of the hole to cover any sharp projections and stones. A butyl pond liner, 7 by 7 metres was then laid in the hole and clamped at the top edges to stop it falling in. This prevents water draining through the pool structure which would accelerate any cooling. A further 20mm of blinding was laid on this pond liner followed by 100mm Xpool insulation, laid and secured with tape to form a box structure.

4. 200mm depth of concrete (reinforced with glass fibres) was laid on the floor of the pool with a steel-reinforcing cage included. Upright reinforcing rods were positioned within this concrete for the breeze block wall to use. Total volume of concrete was some 2 cubic metres and a further 1 cubic meter was used for the floor of the pump room.

5. Hollow breeze blocks were then used to create the walls of the pool. The pipework for the inlet, outlet, skimmer, lights and vacuum points, as well as the points themselves, were now positioned within and through the blockwork. These pipes were fed to the area to be used for the pump room. Care was taken to ensure all joints were very tight before the blockwork was filled with concrete. The internal of the pool was then cement plastered with 6 inch radius fillets in the wall corners.

6. The brickwork for the small wall to take a conservatory was now constructed around the perimeter of the pool

7. Drainage channels for any water splashed out of the pool were placed at either side and at the front of the pool. These channels were attached to small pipes running into the pump room. A 10mm concrete surround to the pool was angled so that water drains towards these drainage channels. Small holes were pre-drilled into the channels to allow water to ingress from the concrete surface which was then soaked in a good water proofer.

8. SureSet, consisting of a crushed marble and resin mix, was then used to finish the surface to the top of the drainage channels. This is porous, so water will run through to the waterproofed concrete beneath and then to the drainage channels.

9. The pool was then lined with under-felt and foam padding and the liner was then positioned in the pool taking care to avoid any creases or punctures. Holes were cut for the inlet, outlet, vacuum, lights and skimmer ports and their top fittings positioned. A ladder and stainless steel and glass banister were added at the pool side as well as the roller for the pool cover.

10. The pump room area was fitted with the equipment and the pipework as described above.

Managing the Quality of the Pool Water

There are two parts to water quality. The first is the appearance of the water and of the pool structure, which should both be clear and free of obvious particulate matter. The second concerns the amount of invisible contamination within the water, whether that is just dissolved material or living organisms (pathogens). Water will support considerable amounts of contamination.

Removing visible contaminants

Clear and Odourless Water

The pool should always look clear and have no odour. If it is cloudy (i.e. there is a large quantity of microscopic particles in the pool water) then it could mean that the filter or the filter medium needs cleaning. However, there are other reasons, e.g. there may be algae growth, or high levels of metal ions (e.g. copper from the ioniser), or the level of the pH, total alkalinity, stabiliser, calcium hardness, or TDS may be too high; or the chlorine level too low.

Filter the big stuff out

The Mega500 filter tank contains silica-sand media and, as the water flows through it, particles (e.g. plastic, concrete, big bits of bacteria, fungus and algae) are trapped and retained, thus creating clear water in the pool. As more and more particles are retained so the flow of water through the filter slows down and the pressure within the tank increases. The pressure gauge on the top of the filter tank will show this rise.

To remove the particles trapped in the sand, the filter needs to be 'backwashed to waste', typically weekly or more frequently if the pressure gauge indicates it is needed. When you backwash, the flow of water through the filter is reversed. The procedure is:

1. ALWAYS turn the pump off before changing the valve position. The pump operates under E10 and may well be isolated when backwashing is to be done. It will need to be plugged into a socket that is not timed but not turned on.

2. Make sure the waste line is still feeding into the drain (there is no valve) and check that the catchment tank (down the hill) is empty. The outlet tap on the tank should be open so that a slow drain to the ditch takes place.
3. Turn the multiport selector valve (at the front of the filter) clockwise to the backwash position and turn the pump back on. It takes minutes to fill the catchment tank so if the water is very dirty (unlikely) it may need two, or even three, fills.
4. Below the multiport selector valve, there is a sight glass that will show the water as dirty and/or cloudy. Once the water in the sight glass is clear (about 2 minutes) you can stop the backwash by turning off the pump.
5. After the backwash, turn the multiport selector valve clockwise to the rinse position and turn the pump on again. Wait until the water in the sight glass is clear (20-30 seconds normally) then turn the pump off.
6. The multiport selector valve should now be turned clockwise back to filtration. The backwash procedure is now complete. Re-plug the pump to E10 timed.

The pool will have lost up to a foot of water during backwashing and rinsing. To refill:
1. Ensure the pump is off so that there is no competition between the pump and the mains water.
2. Open water main valve (number 13) and wear the valve opener on a cord around your neck (or use a timer)to remind you that it is on.

It takes about two hours to fill the pool from the bottom of the JetVag fascia to the middle of the skimmer mouth. It is very easy to forget that the valve is open and the pool is filling! Use the necklace. Although backwashing the filter removes caught debris, it doesn't fully clean the silica-sand medium. To maintain the filter's efficiency, it should be chemically cleaned annually using a filter-cleansing product (e.g. Blue Horizons Filter Cleaner).

Some debris may be too small to be captured by the filter and if the water becomes cloudy a coagulant (flocculent) can be used. This causes the particles to clump together becoming large enough to be caught or to be vacuumed up from the pool bottom. These particles may be algae. It should be unlikely for algae to be a problem since the pool is internal, but outside this property there are high amounts of moss and lichen growth, implying algae spores will be in the air. There are algaecides available to treat algae (Clear 'N Clean).

Some contamination, particularly algae, may not be clearly visible but may be felt on the pool liner, for example. This can be removed by hand with a sponge (but without any cleaning fluid, such as soap) or the sponge could be attached to the vacuum line pole. This moves the contamination into the water where the sanitiser and filter should clear it.

When the backwash starts you may see a white deposit being flushed out immediately from the Mega filter. This is probably calcium or a calcium compound indicating that the chemical balance of the pool is out.

Vacuum the pool floor and walls

When cleaning the walls and floor, do not use sponges and mops with loose fibres or material that will be left in the pool. Similarly, cleaning solutions will contaminate the pool and create foam. A vacuum-cleaner point just below the surface of the pool allows for the vacuuming of the pool bottom and sides. The vacuumed water is sent straight to waste to avoid dirt clogging the filter. Normally up to about a foot of water is removed. The procedure is:

1. Turn the pump off if it is on (during E10 time) and turn off the ASHP and the UV.
2. Re-plug the pump to a socket that is not timed.
3. Unscrew the cap on the vacuum-cleaner point and insert the vacuum-cleaner pipe with its pole and brush attachment. Secure all joints.
4. Close the valve from the skimmer – Valve 1 (so the pump can never suck air).
5. Close the valve from the pool drain output – Valve 2.
6. Turn the Mega500 filter control valve to 'waste' and make sure that the waste line from the filter is feeding to the drain (no valve).
7. Open the valve from the vacuum cleaner point (Valve 3) and turn the pump on.
8. When vacuuming has finished, turn the pump off and turn the filter control back to filter.
9. Close the vacuum-cleaner valve (Valve 3) and refill the pool to half-way up the skimmer.
10. Open the valve from the pool output ports (Valve 1) and open the valve from the skimmer (Valve 2).
11. Turn the pump on and re-plug to E10 time control and turn on the ASHP and the UV.

Emptying the pool

If it becomes necessary to empty the pool then using the 'waste' line on the filter is one way to do so. There are also portable fully-submersible pumps that can be dropped into the pool with a long hose to pump water outside the pool room.

Adding water

The volume of the pool water will decrease by evaporation and after vacuuming dirty water into the waste line. The water main is connected through its own valve (number 13) with a one-way valve preventing pool water going into the mains and, more importantly, a one-way valve preventing any water travelling backwards through the pipework towards the main pump. Do not have the main pump on whilst mains water is being added since this will cause back-pressure onto the non-return valves and the pump, as well as competition between water flows.

Algae

Algae do not directly cause disease. It is a plant that turns sunlight and carbon dioxide into a nutrient for bacteria and it feeds on nitrates and phosphates (orthophosphates) in the water. If there is an algae problem it is often visible unlike the pathogens and chemical imbalances discussed later. If this is an indoor pool it should not be troubled with algae but the poolroom is a warm wet environment ideal for algae growth. At least the top-edge of the liner and the pool surround will require cleaning using household bleach. There may also be algae that are not visible, as well as spores, present in the filter or elsewhere in the system.

Unchecked algae growth can turn the swimming pool cloudy or makes the pool water green and results in bad odours and tastes as well as slime on the pool walls. Black algae is more difficult to control than green or blue-green algae and can also harm the pool's walls and floor. If there are algae present in the pool water, the chlorine will be used up rapidly trying to combat its growth. This process has a tendency to raise the pH, thus decreasing the efficiency of the remaining free chlorine. Adequate levels of free chlorine will prevent algae from growing out of control. When algae growth is noticed, it requires harsh treatment; usually shock treatment with chlorine or an algaecide is recommended. UV, which this pool uses, may be a better way of killing algae as it passes under the light, but will not stop algae formation.

A typical algaecide (Clear 'N Clean) contains copper sulphate pentahydrate, so copper levels will be raised. Algaecides do not kill bacteria, only the algae the bacteria feed upon, so chlorine must still be added. If there is dark staining at the surface level (particularly in the skimmer, or on grey hair) then that is likely to have been caused by the excess copper introduced by the algaecide. Pool experts often recommend the use of algaecides or chlorine shock but they are usually working with large commercial pools.

When algae are destroyed, they release the nitrates and phosphates they consumed back into the water. Removing nitrates (including nitrites which easily convert to nitrates) and particularly phosphates from the water should destroy all the algae by removing its food source. However, levels 'less than 100 ppb' (i.e. 0.1 ppm) for phosphates are mentioned in the literature, which is difficult to measure let alone achieve. Similarly, nitrates should be maintained at below 25ppm (50ppm, UK water regulations). Phosphates can be precipitated out (and collected in the filter) but high nitrates are more difficult to resolve.

There are algaecides available that will clear the algae but to avoid using them it is necessary to:
1. Treat the rim of the pool and its sides with a bleach/algaecide spray to avoid any growth there, that would then contaminate the pool.
2. Monitor and try to remove nitrates and phosphorous from the pool.
3. Maintain a chorine level that will sanitise the pool and destroy algae.
4. Add enzymes that remove by-products by converting them to CO_2 and H_2O to ensure that the chlorine can concentrate on sanitising the pool.

Removing invisible contaminants and Sanitising the Pool

Clean the People

Clear pool water and clean pool walls do not mean the pool water is 'clean'. Water contains pathogens that are not visible as well as the nutrients that provide food for those pathogens. There are also dissolved solids (chemicals) that may damage the pool structure, piping or equipment. These are all too small for the filter to trap. Of primary concern are the pathogens and their nutrients, and since bathers introduce most of these, they (the bathers) need cleaning before entry. Have a shower to remove sweat, make-up, body butter, hair products etc., as well as clean all orifices, including the nose. Long hair should be in a cap. The pool has a light (and exceptionally clean) 'bather load' compared to public pools.

Balancing the Pool Chemistry

Establishing and keeping the correct water chemical balance is important for many reasons including bather safety and comfort, chemical efficiency, protection of the fabric of the pool and the equipment, water appearance, as well as making it easier to clean the pool. The following is a discussion of what to monitor in the chemistry of the pool water as well as how to measure and to adjust the balances of the various chemicals. The appendices may help in understanding the physical chemistry involved and its terms and units. There is no doubt that pool water chemistry is complicated. Whilst the impact of some of the factors such as temperature and pH are obvious, others, such as the dissociation chemistry and the chemical reactivity involved, are not. The discussion that follows is intended to inform the layman and not the chemical engineer. However, it may be worth referring to appendix 1 for some physical chemistry points.

In a public pool the volume of water is relatively large (say, 200,000 litres) compared to this pool (10,000 litres). This shouldn't give rise to any fundamental difference in the chemistry of the pool, but the amounts of chemical used are considerably smaller and need to be measured more accurately. Changes caused by their addition are likely to take place faster and, without taking care, the stability may be more difficult to maintain.

There are four stages of monitoring and maintaining the pool chemistry that are discussed in detail in this section.
1. Temperature, pH, ORP, TDS - a quick check 'every day or so'.
2. Free Chlorine, Total Chlorine and chloramines, check every fortnight or month but especially if ORP is <650ppm or pH is outside 7.0 to 7.8.
3. Calcium Hardness, Total Alkalinity and the LSI, check every month.
4. Copper, Phosphates, Nitrates, check every month

When balanced, the regular addition of chlorine should maintain the ORP at the correct level for the protection of swimmers from pathogens. It is the oxidation potential, which comes from the chlorine, that is important, since chemical imbalances can prevent the chlorine from working even though the amount present is correct. The pH will creep-up because the added chemicals delivering the chlorine are net alkaline and this may require adjustment (with pH minus) every fortnight or so. Stage 2 allows for the accurate measurement of chlorine to ensure sufficient oxidant is present and that there are not excessive chloramines. Stage 3 looks at the key long-term factors of hardness and alkalinity that, if out of balance (LSI), will eventually cause serious corrosion of, or deposits on, the pool and its equipment. Stage 4 looks at contaminants that are naturally present in water and that can be dangerous if excessive (e.g. metals) or can foster the production of food for pathogens (e.g. phosphates)

The pH of the Water

This is the most important factor on the chemistry of a pool. (pH stands for the **p**otential of **H**ydrogen and is the log of the hydrogen ion concentration.) It is the indicator of the level of acidity or alkalinity that a bather is being exposed to and the potency of other chemical additions depends critically upon pH. The reactions resulting from chemical additions will progress according to the various reactive natures of all the different chemical ions in the pool – at the specific pH and temperature. Change the pH and the balance will change.

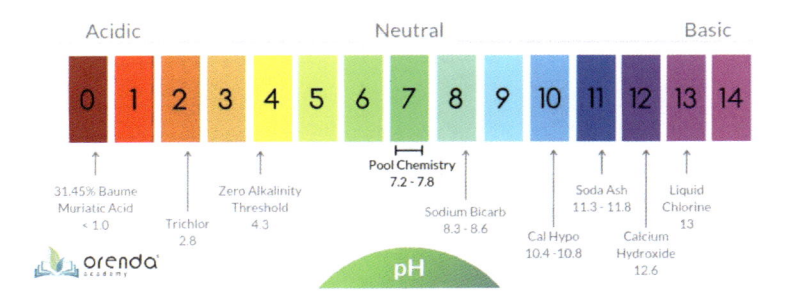

As illustrated in the graph the pH is very dependent upon temperature, for example, a pH of 7.5 at 0°C will fall below 7 at 25°C.

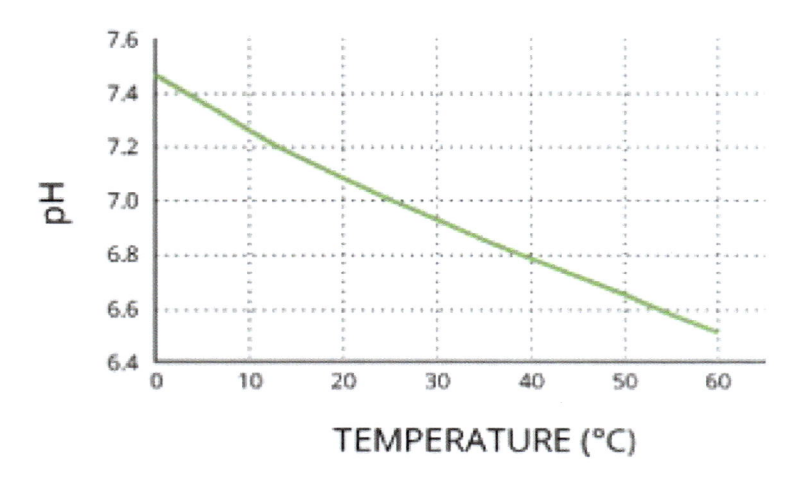

At a pH of 7.0 the water is neutral, with the active oxidising (acidic) ions balanced by the reducing (alkaline or basic) ions. A pH of 7.4 (+/- 0.2) is required – slightly alkaline – for sanitation using chlorine. If it is too low (acidic) then there is the possibility of etching or staining of surfaces, skin and eye irritation, as well as damage to equipment caused by the acidic water. If the pH is too high (alkaline) then scale (calcium carbonate) formation may be encouraged as well as calcification in the filter, cloudy water, drying of the bather's skin and a noticeable reduction in the effectiveness of chlorine.

The pH will change naturally, depending on the temperature, as, for example carbon dioxide is dissolved from the air and seeks an equilibrium. In this case carbonic acid, H_2CO_3, at a low pH of about pH 5, the bicarbonate ion, $H(CO_3)^{1-}$ which peaks at about pH 8, after which is replaced by the carbonate ion $(CO_3)^{2-}$. The addition of chemicals for sanitation and balance can significantly alter the pH as well.

Chlorine

There is no simple measure or mechanism to monitor pathogens in water, so the maintenance of a certain level of sanitiser is necessary. All of the other chemicals are added to ensure the sanitiser operates effectively, to remove the residue of sanitation and other organic matter and to balance the chemical contents of the pool for bather safety and comfort. Along with contamination from users, these additions lead to the increase of the Total Dissolved Solids (TDS, discussed later), which can make it progressively more difficult to maintain a chemical balance.

A sanitation programme ensures that the pool water is healthy by killing microbes that are pathogens (bacteria and virus) and by neutralising organic matter (urine, algae, etc.) that is potential food for the pathogens. It does this by oxidation – the addition of a negative ion. Chlorine is especially valuable as a sanitiser since pathogens are not able to develop immunity to it. (However, cryptosporidium is a particularly hard bug even for chlorine to kill.) Note that there are microbe testing kits available if there are concerns about bacterial infection of the pool.

Bromine is an alternative sanitiser that remains active longer than chlorine (and therefore less is required) and is particularly appropriate for high temperature pools/hot tubs. It doesn't dissolve or oxidise as well as chlorine and can leave the pool cloudy but it doesn't produce the same odour from its by-products and is more effective than chlorine at high pH levels. In practice some commercial products are a mixture of bromine and chlorine compounds.

The 'chlorine' used is normally Sodium Hypochlorite (NaOCl). In this pool Calcium Hypochlorite Ca(OCl)$_2$ is used since this can be obtained without Cyanuric Acid stabiliser (discussed later). The chlorine becomes ionised into positive sodium or calcium ions and hypochlorous acid (HOCl) and the less active hypochlorite ions (OCl). It is the latter two acids (particularly HOCl because it is more reactive) that oxidise molecules on the cells of pathogens, killing them. The proportion of these two is shown for pH below:

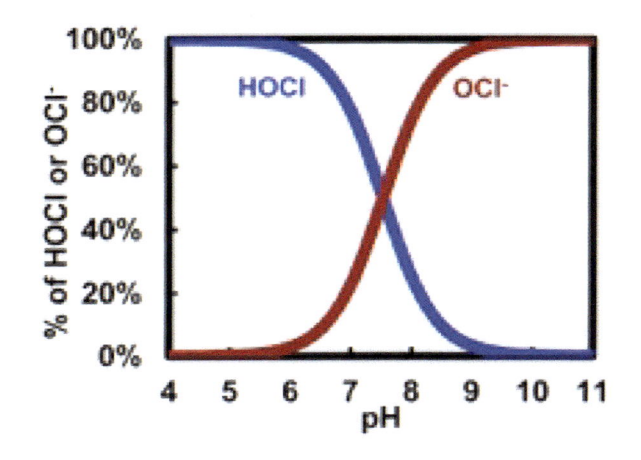

Commercial pools maintain the chlorine level at about 2 to 4ppm of pool water but with using UV it should be possible to hold the chlorine level at 1ppm or below in this pool.

There are three aspects to the chlorine in a pool:

1. 'Free', (also called 'available' or 'residual') chlorine is the amount of chlorine in the pool that is available to sanitise (disinfect) the water.
2. Combined chlorines (mono, di-, tri-chloramines) are the bad-smelling and irritating compounds that are the products of chlorine disinfection. These also have some disinfection ability and they slowly evaporate.
3. Total chlorine is the sum of free and combined chlorine compounds.

When chlorine is initially added to water it undergoes a fast reaction with any contaminants, e.g. ammonia NH_3 (from urine). This results in the formation of chloramines as the free chlorine is converted to combined chlorine. The chlorine is further used-up as it kills organisms – which is the real intention in adding it to the pool – or as it combines with other chemicals.

Where the literature states it, the level of chloramines should be maintained below 0.5ppm. To achieve this, it may become necessary to run off a quantity of pool water as described in the Total Dissolved Solids section.

The effectiveness of the free chlorine depends upon the pH, **so the pH must be adjusted before the chlorine**. When the pH is 8.0 the chlorine is only 20% effective and at a pH of 8.5 the chlorine is only 8% effective. Chlorine becomes 'overactive' when the pH is lower than 7.0 and the acidic water may cause damage to metals (pumps) and plastics (pool liner and pipework).

If the chlorine level should keep falling (chlorine demand) then it is being used up and needs slow and careful replacement to avoid excess. It is usual to add a set amount and wait 24 hours to see the effect and to keep doing this until the chlorine level stops falling.

You can 'shock' the pool by putting in about 10 times the concentration of the Free Chlorine to clear the chlorine demand, but it is extreme dosing of the pool. In this case Calcium Hypochlorite, $Ca(OCl)_2$ is used (as the source of chlorine) but the reason for its selection is not clear from any of the literature. It is probably because it is sold without Cyanuric acid (CYA) but it may also be because it has a higher dissociation and therefore a larger amount of HOCl acid is produced, or there is more (twice as much) HOCl for a given quantity of anion (Ca) – so you add less calcium. Rather than shocking the pool, it may be better to run off a quantity of water, since every time you add chemicals directly you increase the Total Dissolved Solids (TDS).

The term Chlorine Demand is often used to describe the situation where chlorine appears to be disappearing from the pool. This is misleading because chlorine will always be disappearing (chlorine and chloramine evaporation, chlorine neutralisation of bather load, UV action, etc.). Sometimes it is used to describe the initial period in an untreated pool when the chlorine is quickly used up and sometimes it is used even when there is plenty of free chlorine. In the case of this pool the term will be used to describe the rate at which the free chlorine falls from the time chlorine is added to the time when its ppm level falls to the low point again. This is discussed in more detail later.

In removing contaminants in the water, the free chlorine oxidises them and the actual oxidising potential of the water can be measured, in mV, by an ORP (Oxidation/Reduction Potential) meter. Maintaining an ORP of 750 mV at a pH of 7.4 by using chlorine should ensure a well-sanitised pool.

Enzymes

It is the very effective oxidising capability of chlorine (i.e. HOCl) that kills bacteria by stripping electrons from the cell's surface or by damaging its proteins (human cells produce HOCl to attack invading pathogens). However, chlorine will oxidise not only the bacteria but also other chemicals in the water, i.e. residual non-living organics from dead algae and bacteria, sweat, as well as cosmetics etc. This is not only a waste of the chlorine but leaves chloramines behind encouraging more chlorine demand. By adding enzymes these organics can be converted to carbon dioxide and water, leaving the chlorine to focus upon bacteria.

Practical Pool Management or "So, where is all the chlorine going?"

The ideal would be a pool with an ORP of 750mV (at a pH of 7.4) achieved by adding chlorine, with the UV/ioniser operational and the TDS below 500ppm. In practice it is to be expected that the free chlorine level (and the related ORP) will simply fall as pathogens, algae and bather load are destroyed. However, the chlorine additions required to maintain the free chlorine level are often larger and more frequent than anticipated. This highlights how difficult it can be to overcome bacterial or algae growth rates and additions from bathers as well as the natural evaporation of free chlorine and chloramines.

The normal removal of chloramines is achieved by adding more chlorine, transforming mono-chloramine to the volatile di-chloramine and then to the most volatile (and smelly) tri-chloramine. If chlorine is not added in sufficient quantity and fast enough then the growth rates of bacteria and algae will cause a steady build up (and slow removal) of chloramines and it will therefore be impossible to maintain a level of (free) chlorine. The literature tries to illustrate what actually happens using graphs such as the following.

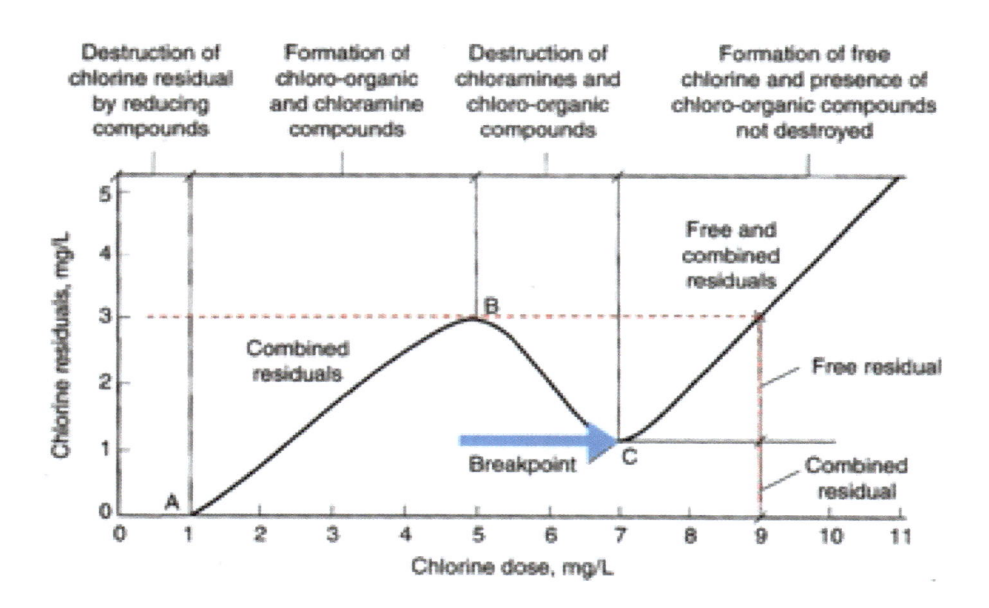

The x-axis here is confusing. It implies that, for example, adding 5mg/L (ppm) of chlorine will enable the point 'B' of total chlorine to be reached, or by adding, say, 1mg/L continuously you will proceed along the curve to beyond point 'C'. In practice, much larger doses of chlorine are applied on an irregular basis – often days in between. However, this is a useful graph to explain the **breakpoint principal** describing the break-away from the battle with pathogens and excess chloramines.

The y-axis shows the residual chlorine and chloramine (Total Chlorine). At low levels of added chlorine, it is quickly used up and the algae and bacteria will continue to multiply to point 'A'. At higher chlorine doses more chloramines are produced and the level of total chlorine rises to a peak ('B'). If insufficient chlorine is added then the level falls back and, again, algae and bacteria will multiply.

Provided enough chlorine is added then the chloramines are slowly removed until a breakpoint is reached ('C') when the chloramine production has been largely overcome. At this point the amount of free chlorine begins to rise with additional added chlorine, although some residual chloramines will remain. The speed with which the breakpoint is reached is important in order to overcome the growth rates of bacteria and algae – and this is the main point of such graphs. Chloramines, along with any additional bacteria, algae and bather load, will continue to use up free chlorine so it is necessary to continue adding low levels after reaching 'C'.

To try to identify how best to do this, the free chlorine, total chlorine, and chloramine levels (in ppm) have been monitored daily, as shown in the following graph. The chloramines can be seen to be rising and falling but remain near 0.5ppm. Free and total chlorine appear to fall at the same rate of about 0.5ppm per day.

The chlorine dosage depends on the actual concentration in the 'calcium hypochlorite' supplied (see the side of the container), which is not just pure calcium hypochlorite (this is discussed further later on). The additions noted here are weights of the powder from the container used. Whilst these raise the free chlorine, at low quantities the improvement is not proportional. The rate of fall of chlorine appears to be the same but the increase produced by the lowest levels of added chlorine is less. This maybe because of pH variance or the impact of other chemicals at low chlorine concentration or that the smaller additions of chlorine find it harder to overcome the chloramine build-up.

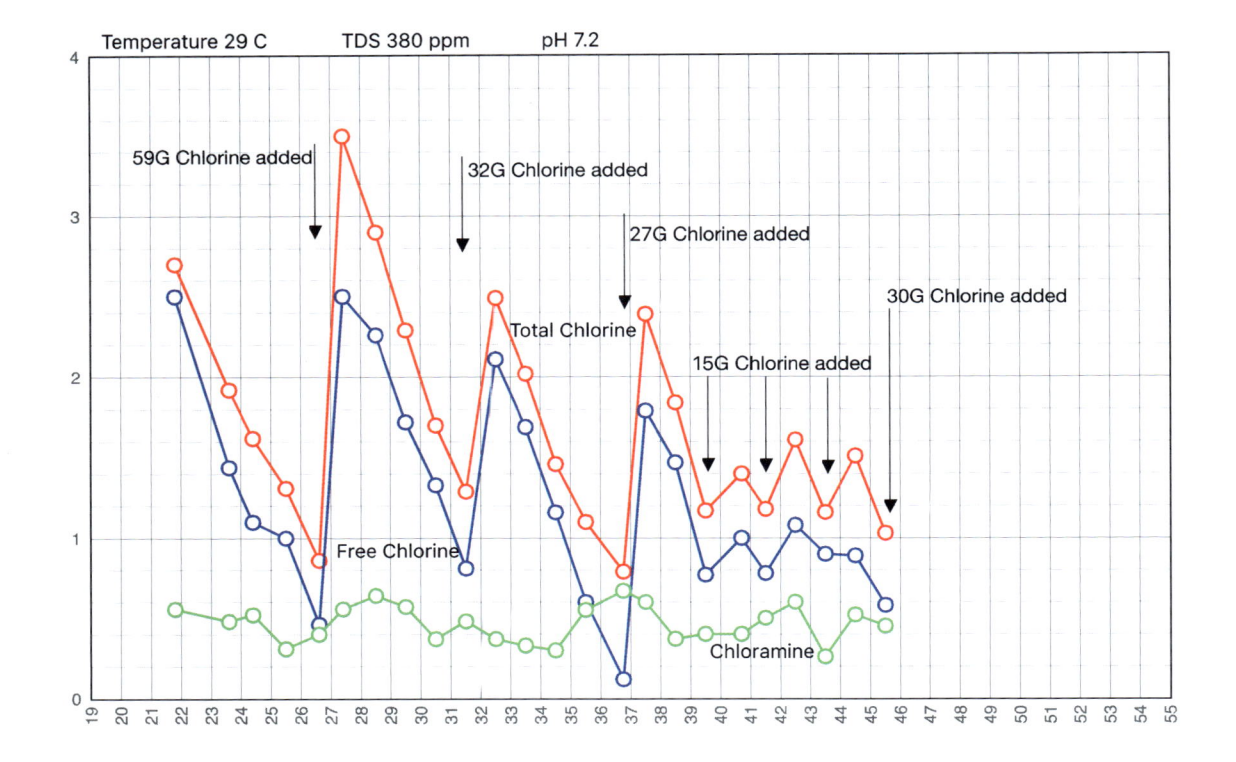

Interestingly, the graph also shows that chlorine should have been added on day 35 and that the chloramines began to rise above 0.5 when the free chlorine fell to below 0.5. This is the fallback towards the breakpoint 'C' discussed above. As a result, a dosage of 27g (from the Calcium Hypochlorite supplier's container) was added on day 36. The discipline (for this pool) of adding 15g every two days would therefore seem appropriate to maintaining an average free chlorine level of 1ppm. Alternatively, the addition of about 30g every 4 days would still maintain free chlorine within acceptable boundaries.

What is not shown clearly in this graph is the fact that pH had to be adjusted over the time period. This is because the 'Calcium Hypochlorite' supplied, i.e. the total contents of the container, are alkaline. This may seem strange, since it is intended to produce HOCl and OCl acids, but it is correct and the pH will increase slowly with each addition. An increase of about 0.2 pH for each 30g addition occurred. To correct this the addition of pH decreaser (Sodium Bisulphate) was regularly done some hours after the chlorine adjustment.

Algaecides, Nitrates and Phosphates

To ensure that the chlorine is free to focus upon bacteria the prior removal of algae with algaecides or by 'shock' may be necessary as described above. Similarly, the removal of nitrates and phosphates is desirable to remove this food source for the algae.

It is often recommended that nitrates (which term is used to cover nitrites as well), should be removed from the pool by replacing some of the water. That is not satisfactory as the source of the nitrates is usually the tap water itself. Ion exchange and osmosis equipment are unrealistically expensive and the removal of nitrates is still a work-in-progress. Nitrates may also be produced, instead of tri-chloramines, as the chlorine burns off ammonia.

The phosphate level is usually very low and is often described in parts per billion. Pool companies talk about maintaining levels well below 0.5 ppm but UK water companies add 1 to 2 ppm partly to stop lead pipes dissolving. This is a key food for algae so it is important to make it as low as possible. The compound involved in removing phosphates is a lanthanide, which coats the filter sand and reacts with any phosphates, extracting them from the water. Back-washing is then required to remove the resulting compounds. Measure the water going into your pool before deciding on any treatment.

Cyanuric Acid (CYA)

CYA is also referred to as 'stabiliser' or 'conditioner' and is added to external pools to prevent the loss of free chlorine under the influence of the sun, i.e. UV. It should not be needed for internal pools.

The CYA molecule binds weakly to the free chlorine molecule and shields it from the UV. The weak bond ensures that, when the level of chlorine that is not bound to CYA falls below the equilibrium point, more chlorine is released from CYA. By partially locking away chlorine, CYA causes the suppression of the oxidisation potential and a high concentration of CYA can withhold the chlorine so well that it is not be available for sanitising the pool at all. Less than 15ppm is recommended to be present in a pool.

It is not intended to use CYA in this pool despite the fact that the use of UV ioniser as the prime sanitiser may cause a loss of chlorine. Unfortunately, the usual source of chlorine

(Sodium Hypochlorite) is sold with CYA already mixed in as Sodium Hypochloroisocyanurate/Dichloroisocyanurate/Trichloroisocyanurate. Calcium Hypochlorite ('shock') is non-stabilised (i.e. no CYA) and is to be preferred.

The UV-C Ioniser

The amount of chlorine required to sanitise the pool is significantly reduced by using a UV-C ioniser, but it still needs to be monitored and maintained at a certain level. Normally the amount of chlorine is specified at 2 to 4ppm of pool water. Using the UV-C ioniser means that the target chlorine level may be reduced since sanitation is achieved by:

1. UV irradiation (210 to 310nM) of an organism's DNA causing it to die or at least not to be able to reproduce, at 30mJ/cm^2. To be most effective the UV must be broad spectrum in order to prevent DNA self-repair by the microbes. Up to 80% disinfection can be achieved with the UV radiation independently.
2. The ioniser (if activated) releasing trace amounts (to be managed at 0.5ppm) of copper ions into the water that attach to bacterial surface proteins eventually killing them. Ionisation purifies the water very slowly. Up to 20% disinfection can be achieved with the copper ioniser independently.
3. In addition to the disinfection of the water, UV also affects the chloramines that are the by-products of the chlorine sanitation. The nitrogen-chlorine or the nitrogen-hydrogen bonds of the chloramines are broken producing hydroxyl (OH) radicals, oxidising the chloramines. High energy UV (60mJ/cm^2) is required for this action.

The graph shows the UV radiation from a typical UV lamp with the corresponding relative germicidal effectiveness.

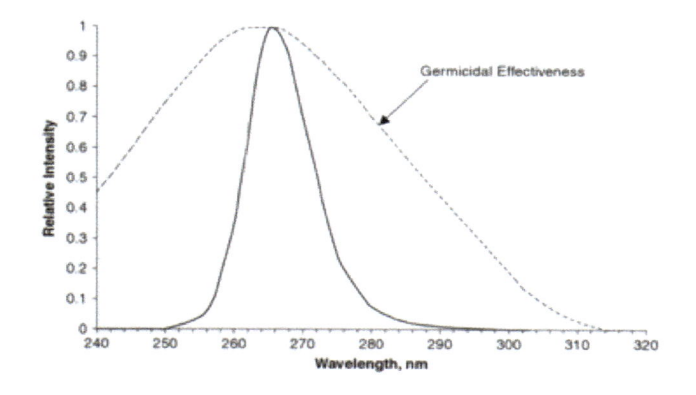

In combination, the UV-C Ioniser could be thought to achieve much of the necessary disinfection of the water, but it does not produce a 'chemical-treatment-free' pool. It is still necessary to add chlorine since:

1. Not all of the bacteria are in the water all the time
2. Bathers will introduce further contamination
3. Some bacteria will self-repair
4. There is a lag before water passes under the UV-C ioniser
5. Copper ions act slowly
6. UV light actually breaks down some dissociated chlorine (HOCl and OCl).

The advantage of UV-C ioniser is that it should be possible to reduce and maintain chlorine levels to at, or below, 1ppm.

Hardness and Total Alkalinity

Water dissolves 'stuff' – mainly the calcium carbonate and nitrates in the ground through which it passes. In addition, water supplies are treated with, for example, chlorine (to 'kill bugs') and phosphates (to protect pipework from corrosion). Dissolved carbon dioxide from the air also contributes significantly to the alkalinity of water. The reactivity of each of these chemicals depends upon factors such as the pH of the water and the temperature.

Calcium carbonate is particularly important because it is the primary source of the 'total alkalinity' and the 'hardness' of the water. The latter is a measure of the calcium (and in smaller quantities, magnesium, sodium and potassium) in the water, whereas the total alkalinity is a measure of the carbonate (and in smaller quantities, hydroxide, bicarbonate, etc.)

If the water contains a great deal of calcium carbonate (i.e. it is 'hard') then there will be a tendency for the calcium to precipitate out on to surfaces (including the filter medium) and the water may become cloudy. It may also reduce the effectiveness of the sanitiser. Conversely, if there is little calcium carbonate (i.e. it is 'soft') then the water will dissolve it (or equivalent compounds) from the structure of the pool, resulting in etching of surfaces, staining or the production of foam. (Note that if the calcium hardness falls this could be due to calcium combining with phosphates and that implies the possible presence of algae).

The technical measure for water's hardness is the mmols/Lt of calcium ions. However, this is more usefully expressed as the ppm of calcium carbonate dissolved in the water that would be required to produce the mmols/Lt of calcium ions.

The use of Calcium Hypochlorite as the sanitiser will add calcium as well as chlorine. It is estimated that 0.8ppm of calcium is added for every 1ppm of free chlorine produced, and whilst the chlorine is used up and leaves the pool, the calcium will remain. At the dosages discussed above, to maintain 1ppm of chlorine, the calcium concentration will have been raised by about 24ppm in three months compared to a target of 220ppm for hardness. This slow increase in calcium will become a factor in maintaining balance.

Total Alkalinity is not the same as 'alkaline' on the pH scale, which defines whether something is acid or alkaline. Total alkalinity is a measurement of the concentration of all alkaline substances dissolved in the water. When a solution has a high total alkalinity, it means that it is more able to 'buffer' the addition of acid so that the pH does not change much. Add acid to pure water and it will immediately show a low pH. Add it to high total alkalinity water and it will take much more acid before the pH changes. Total alkalinity is a measure of this 'buffering capacity'.

Just as for hardness, the measure for water's total alkalinity is reported as the ppm of calcium carbonate dissolved in the water that would be required to produce the particular mmols/Lt of carbonate ions.

If the pH is difficult to set then the water's total alkalinity is the likely cause. If the total alkalinity is too low then the pH will fluctuate and it will be difficult to maintain the ideal level. On the other hand, if it is too high then the pH can be difficult to change and may keep rising.

The use of Calcium Hypochlorite as the sanitiser has a further consequence. The product supplied contains calcium chloride and combined water as well as the active ingredient and the product as a whole is alkaline. When dissolved in water it reacts to produce the chlorine acids. However, the net effect can be to raise the pH without raising the total alkalinity. Yet adding Sodium Bisulphate to lower the pH should also lower the total alkalinity. In practice, by adding small quantities of the appropriate chemicals, waiting a day and measuring again will enable a good balance to be struck.

The ranges required for balanced water are:
Hardness: 200ppm (water corrosive) to 275ppm (scale formation, ineffective chlorine)
Total Alkalinity: 80ppm (pH unstable) to 150ppm (scale formation, pH too stable).

However, the use of ranges for each chemical ignores the fact that variations in the hardness and alkalinity (coupled with the levels of pH, temperature and all the other various dissolved solids) interact with one another to produce a certain level of chemical balance or 'saturation' in the water. What is really required is to ensure that the actual chemical balance does not cause corrosion or scale formation. This is resolved by using the Langelier Saturation Index (see Appendix 2 for the theory).

Langelier Saturation Index (LSI) – The Practice

The LSI is an equilibrium model derived from the theoretical concept of saturation and provides an indicator of the degree of saturation of water with respect to calcium carbonate. It determines if water is corrosive (i.e. it will dissolve calcium carbonate as it is under-saturated, negative LSI), balanced (0.0 LSI), or scale forming (i.e. calcium carbonate precipitates out because the water is over-saturated, positive LSI). It simply indicates the driving force for scale formation or corrosion. Making changes to pH or temperature will change the index, and they are referred to as master variables.

Calculating the LSI identifies the necessary changes to the hardness and alkalinity in order to bring the LSI to zero. Whilst it is not strictly necessary, it is reasonable to make changes so that they are also within the individual 'ideal ranges' for hardness or alkalinity mentioned above. It is possible to calculate the amounts of each chemical addition required to correct the LSI from first principles (see appendix) but those nice people at ORENDA have kindly produced an app for this. However, the corrective dosages recommended by them refer to their chemicals from their containers and it is necessary to estimate the equivalents of the chemicals required from the details provided by your suppliers and this is always clearly stated on the side of the tub.

Total Dissolved Solids (TDS)

TDS is the total of dissolved solids in the water including; minerals, the chemicals that have been added and reaction products, (i.e. chloramines, any stabilisers (e.g. CYA), metal ions, carbonates, bicarbonates, hydroxides, etc.), dissolved biological materials, and dissolved elements of plastic, metal, concrete, etc. TDS must be maintained below 1000 ppm. (TDS, like calcium hardness, needs further restriction if an electrical heater is to be used.) Correcting problems with the pool, as well as sanitisation, will change its chemical balance and increase the TDS. The regular replacing of some of the pool water will reduce the TDS, and this will be partially achieved by the regular backwash cycle and vacuuming.

Balancing the Pool Chemistry – Measurements

See the flow chart in Appendix 4 for an idealised sequence of testing and appendix 6 for the meters used. Before taking measurements or if measurements are way out of expectation then the meters may well need cleaning and recalibrating.

Measure the temperature, pH and ORP daily. It is worth creating a graph, based on the chlorine levels each day, as shown earlier but when a regular regime of adding chlorine is established the measurement of free and total chlorine can be delayed to every fortnight or even later. At that time measure the TDS, Phosphate, Nitrate, Copper, Hardness and Alkalinity. If these show signs of being out of balance make the necessary corrections and monitor more regularly until they settle down.

The pH of the Water

Use the meter to measure the pH. A pH of 7.4 (+/- 0.2) is required – slightly alkaline – for sanitisation using chlorine.

Temperature

Use a meter to measure the temperature to check that the ASHP is working correctly.

ORP

Use the (Hanna) ORP meter to determine that the oxidation potential is between 650 and 750 mV. You may need to measure the ORP and the free chlorine at the same time to obtain a comparison between them. That should provide confidence that you know the free chlorine level and it is giving adequate oxidation.

Chlorine

Use the Hanna titration test kits to measure the free chlorine and total chlorine levels. With the UV-C ioniser active the chlorine level should be maintained at, or near 1ppm. (The ORP is the key measure since it is the oxidation capability that is important, rather than the amount of chlorine.) Correct the level slowly leaving 24 hours before taking the next measurement.

Nitrates and Phosphates

Use the test kits to determine the levels. Nitrates should be maintained below 25 ppm and phosphates below 2 ppm.

Hardness

Use the titration test kit to measure the hardness. This is the total of all the mineral salts dissolved in the water and should be maintained in the range of 200 to 275 ppm.

Total Alkalinity

Use the titration test kit to measure the alkalinity. This is the measure of the alkali, i.e. bicarbonates, carbonates and hydroxides, present in the pool and should be maintained at 80 to 150ppm in order for the pH to be stable.

LSI

Having gathered all the above measurements, the LSI can be found using the ORENDA app that also indicates the appropriate changes to make to rebalance the pool water.

Copper

Use a simple colour change test strip to ensure copper levels are well below 0.7ppm.

Total Dissolved Solids (TDS)

Use the meter to measure the TDS, which should be maintained below 1000ppm. If it is high, say above 500ppm, then it is necessary to replace some of the pool water. This will be partially achieved by the regular backwash cycle or vacuuming.

Balancing the Pool Chemistry – Applying chemicals

Notes:

1. **Never add water to the powder (or liquid) chemical as this may cause an aggressive exothermic reaction throwing the liquid back at you. Always <u>add the powder to a full container of water</u> **
2. It is important to buy chemicals that are specifically designed for swimming pools, as sometimes any 'impurities' may be inappropriate for a pool.
3. Always check the instructions on the side of the container. This should tell you the actual amount of chemical from the container to add to an amount of pool water in order to achieve a specific dosage of the active chemical required. The latter will only be one of the chemicals in the container. The amounts noted below (using the term 'typical') are examples of dose rates from various suppliers, brochures and guides and make assumptions about the chemical balance existing in the pool as well as concentrations of the active ingredient supplied. The amount to add should always be calculated from the instructions on the container.
4. The actual amount of active ingredient in the container may be surprising low (and sometimes not declared) e.g. 60% in the case of chlorine products. This may be because of the manufacturing or purification processes or because of the inclusion of other chemicals for long-term stability of the active ingredient whilst in storage.
5. With some of the chemical rebalancing it is only possible to make a guess at the amount to be added to the pool. Make this amount small and re-measure. 24 hours is a reasonable time to wait between adding a chemical and measuring the effect.
6. The instructions on the side of the container will also tell you the dangers associated with the chemical and the action to take if there is an accident.

7. Pour the solution in front of the water inlet port to the pool and always ensure the pump is running for at least an hour after chemicals are added to enable good mixing. If you dose the pool in the evening then it should be ready to use the next day.
8. A spreadsheet is available (appendix 5) for recording the values of the different readings and the chemicals added, to enable long-term monitoring of the pool water.

pH 7.4 +/- 0.2.

- If it is below 7.2, add 'pH increaser' = Sodium Carbonate (soda ash)
- If it is above 7.6, add 'pH decreaser' = Sodium Bisulphate (dry acid)

'Typically': (i.e. from experience with chemicals purchased)
To increase pH by 0.2, add 100g of sodium carbonate to the pool.
To decrease pH, add 100g of sodium bisulphate **to** a bucket of pool water (never add the water to the acid) and slowly (over days) add the solution to the pool whilst monitoring the pH.

The Addition of Enzymes and the Removal of Phosphates

Adding enzymes will save chlorine being used up on impurities (e.g. algae residues) and make it easier to maintain the chlorine level. **Typically** the addition of 250 mL is required for this pool. Likewise, the appropriate amount of phosphate remover will starve any algae and save further chlorine. Note that backwashing is then required.

Maintaining the Free Chlorine and Total Chlorine Levels

With the UV-C ioniser active, the chlorine level should be maintained at below 1ppm. Correct the level slowly, leaving 24 hours between each addition. This pool of 10,000 litres requires 10g of actual free chlorine to be at 1ppm. Check the instructions on the side of the container. **Typically** this will say 'Calcium Hypochlorite' – to increase the chlorine level by 1ppm add 150g per 100M^3 i.e. 100,000L. That is 15g, of the actual compounds in the container, for this 10,000L pool to achieve 1ppm free chlorine increase. As can be seen from the graph above, experience indicates that twice that may be needed in practice.

The literature often states that total chlorine is as a proxy for free chlorine since combined chlorine (chloramines) should be low. In practice the difference between the two can be as much as 0.5ppm. If the test for total chlorine is vastly out of line then there is an excessive quantity of chloramines present (which will smell) and the Total Dissolved Solids may also be high.

Hardness and Total Alkalinity

Targeting the total hardness at 240ppm and the total alkalinity at 120ppm and using the ORENDA LSI app will provide the actual amounts required to rebalance. Independent of that app, if the total hardness is too low then, **typically**, to increase it by 10ppm add 150g of calcium chloride for this pool. If the total hardness is too high, then water should be replaced (see TDS).

Typically the total alkalinity level may be raised by 10ppm by adding 140g of sodium bicarbonate and lowered by 10ppm by adding 20g of sodium bisulphate. It may take days for the total alkalinity to change completely after making additions.

Copper

If copper levels are high use a typical 'No More Metals' additive and backwash.

Total Dissolved Solids (TDS)

This may be measured using the meter and should be maintained below 1000ppm. Electronic measurement (+/- 10% accuracy) measures the electrical conductivity and applies a 'correction factor'. To reduce a high level of TDS, flush out a quantity of the water (say a foot of depth) and replace it with fresh water.

Microbe Testing

There are microbe test kits available (e.g. Watersafe) if you feel it is necessary to test for any reason. If they prove positive contact the water board and ask where to get testing done.

The Chemicals Used

1. Blue Horizons Filter Cleaner (to clean the filter medium)

2. Gold Horizons Enzyme ([ORENDA](#) products are currently USA only)
3. Clear 'N Clean algaecide
4. Blue Horizons 'PhosAway'
5. Sodium Carbonate (soda ash) – to increase pH - Na_2CO_3
6. Sodium Bisulphate (dry acid) – to decrease pH - $NaHSO_4$
7. Sodium Bicarbonate - to raise Total Alkalinity (TA) - $NaHCO_3$
8. Sodium Bisulphate (dry acid) – to lower Total Alkalinity (TA) - $NaHSO_4$
9. Calcium Chloride – to increase Total or Calcium Hardness - $CaCl_2$
10. Calcium Hypochlorite – high oxidation potential - chlorine ("shock") – $Ca(ClO)_2$ without CYA or other Stabiliser
11. Sodium dichloroisocyanurate ($C_3Cl_2N_3NaO_3$) or trichloroisocyanurate ($C_3Cl_3N_3O_3$) – chlorine (includes CYA)
12. Sodium Hypochlorite - liquid chlorine additive – (common bleach at 5%) – $NaClO$

Maintenance Sequence

Weekly Maintenance of the Equipment

1. Check all equipment is functioning correctly in the pump room.
2. Visual check for water leaks in the pump room.
3. Check the filter's pressure gauge and the cleanliness of the filter water.
4. Visual check of the cleanliness all of the pool liner and the pool surroundings.

Monthly Maintenance of the Pool Water

As weekly plus:

1. Visual check for electrical cable security.
2. Clean the strainer basket in the pump (& silicone grease the 'O' ring).
3. Clean the strainer basket in the skimmer.
4. Clean the top of the liner and the pool surround with household bleach.
5. Measure the temperature, pH, ORP, TDS and the free chlorine.
6. Measure the Total (Calcium) Hardness and the Total Alkalinity and calculate the LSI.
7. Check the copper concentration with test strip.
8. Make adjustments accordingly.

Annual Maintenance of the Equipment and the Pool

1. Use 'Watersafe' to test for microbes.
2. Clean the filter's media using a filter-cleansing product.
3. The UV lamp should be replaced after a set number of hours e.g. every year.
4. The copper rod of the ioniser can become covered in deposits so it should be cleaned with a copper wire brush after dipping in a cleaner. (To ensure that the ioniser is easy to open next time smear its 'O' rings with silicone grease afterwards.)

Appendices

Appendix 1: Physical Chemistry

To be really clear about chemical additions and balances it is necessary to understand a little physical chemistry, the nomenclature used, the primary chemicals involved and the details of their measurement.

- [For this work, mg/l is equivalent to, ppm, parts per million](). The contaminant or active ingredient ('solute'), in mg, is dissolved in 1 litre of water ('solvent'). Since the density of water is 1g per ml, the solute **in mg** is actually dissolved in 1kg of water. That is equivalent to the solute **in grams** being dissolved in 1000kG of water, or 1 part (1G) in 1 million (1000kG) parts of water. (This neglects the volume of the solute).

- Chemical reactions proceed both backwards and forwards at rates that depend upon factors such as temperature, the pH, the mixture of chemicals in the solution and the contaminants. For example, the pH (which is a measure of the hydrogen ions present) has a dramatic effect on the balance of other chemicals that are in solution as ions or as compounds. The dissociation of Calcium Hypochlorite into Calcium, HOCl and OCl produces ions that are individually more or less reactive depending on temperature. Each chemical ion has a different tendency to react or to dissociate, which is why managing their balance can be difficult.

- pH is the critical factor in pool chemistry. It is a logarithmic scale used to specify the acidity or alkalinity of an aqueous solution. When pH = 7 the water is neither acidic (lower numbers) nor alkaline (higher numbers). (Note that pH is exactly 7 for distilled water since all the dissolved chemicals are left behind in the distillation process.)

- Don't confuse a target ppm (e.g. 1mG/L = 1ppm of chlorine) for the amount of an additive required to be put into the pool. The latter is also often expressed in mG/L e.g. 1.5mG/L of Chlorine (= 15G/10,000L of pool water).

- If the addition of, e.g. chlorine, uses solid (granular) additive, the instruction to use, say, 1G per 1,000L of pool water (i.e. 10G for this pool) is straightforward. However, when adding a chemical that is already dissolved in water the difficulty arises of just how much active chemical in milligrams (the solute) is being input. For example, liquid chlorine is often provided in solutions of various strengths (e.g. 5% (common bleach), 10% or 15%). So, rather than calculate the actual weight of chemical being added, the usual procedure is to add a small amount to try to reach a stable target level over a 24-hour period. This is not ideal, but the type and the quantity of contaminants added by a bather (that have changed the pool's chemical balance) are unknown anyway.

- It is sometimes desirable to know exactly how much chlorine is being added from a liquid chlorine bottle. Expressing the strength as a percentage means that a 15% weight/volume (w/v) solution has been made by dissolving 15G of chlorine to make a total of 100mL of solution. Thus a 15% w/v solution has 15G in 100mL of water and so, in 400ml of 15% chlorine (which is the usual product strength for pools) there is 60g of chlorine. Similarly, 40ml contains 6g.

- To dose the pool from zero chlorine to 1mG/L requires each litre of pool water to contain 1mG. So 10,000 litres requires 10G of chlorine. This amount would be contained in 66mL (6.6 x 1.5 =10G) of 15% w/v liquid chlorine.

Appendix 2: The Theory of The Langelier Saturation Index (LSI)

The Langelier Saturation index (LSI) is an equilibrium model derived from the theoretical concept of saturation and provides an indicator of the degree of saturation of water with respect to calcium carbonate. It determines if water is corrosive (under-saturated, low LSI), balanced, or scale forming (over-saturated, high LSI). It simply indicates the driving force for scale formation in terms of pH as a master variable. Making changes to pH, or temperature, as well as evaporation, will change the index.

LSI is the deviation of the pH from the condition where the water is fully saturated with calcium carbonate. At zero deviation calcium carbonate will neither precipitate out nor be etched into the water.

Calculating the LSI allows changes of hardness, alkalinity or pH to be made that will bring the LSI to zero. Whilst it is not strictly necessary, it is ideal to change the hardness or alkalinity to remain, or return, to being within their ideal ranges.

It is possible to prepare the factors A, B, C, D as a chart to be able to read off values (avoiding the use of log tables) but ORENDA has kindly produced an app for this. It can be used to identify the amount of chemical to add that will change the hardness or the alkalinity to bring the LSI to zero.

LSI is defined as:

    $LSI = pH - pH_s$
    Where:
        pH is the measured water pH
        pH_s is the pH at saturation in calcium carbonate and is defined as:

    $pH_s = (9.3 + A + B) - (C + D)$
    Where:
        $A = (Log_{10} [TDS] - 1) / 10$ (takes ionic strength into account)
        $B = -13.12 \times Log_{10} (°C + 273) + 34.55$ (takes temperature into account)
        $C = Log_{10} [Ca^{2+}$ as $CaCO_3] - 0.4$ (takes hardness into account)

$$D = \text{Log}_{10}[\text{alkalinity as CaCO}_3] \text{ (takes alkalinity into account)}$$

(I cannot find the derivation of this formula.)

If CYA is present then a correction factor needs to be applied to the measured alkalinity, reducing it by about 15%, depending on the pH.

An example of the calculation:
- pH = 7.5
- TDS = 320mg/L
- Hardness = 150mg/L (or ppm) as $CaCO_3$
- Alkalinity = 34mg/L (or ppm) as $CaCO_3$

LSI Formula:
- LSI = pH - pH_s
- pH_s = (9.3 + A + B) - (C + D) where:
    - A = (Log_{10}[TDS] - 1)/10 = 0.15
    - B = -13.12 x Log_{10}(°C + 273) + 34.55 = 2.09 at 25°C and 1.09 at 82°C
    - C = Log_{10}[Ca^{2+} as $CaCO_3$] - 0.4 = 1.78
    - D = Log_{10}[alkalinity as $CaCO_3$] = 1.53
- At 25°C:
- pH_s = (9.3 + 0.15 + 2.09) - (1.78 + 1.53) = 8.2
- LSI = 7.5 - 8.2 = - 0.7
- No Tendency to Scale

- Calculation at 82°C:
- pH_s = (9.3 + 0.15 + 1.09) - (1.78 + 1.53) = 7.2
- LSI = 7.5 - 7.2 = + 0.3
- Slight Tendency to Scale

Appendix 3: Hints and tips on joining pipework.

It is clearly necessary to ensure that all joints are water-tight. This is particularly true where the pipes will be hidden from view.

1. Dry fitting the arrangement of pipes helps to position and size the various pipes BUT the joints are really tight when dry, so sizing the pipework this way can only be approximate.

2. When wet with the Griffin glue, the joints slide very easily. Then the issue becomes to ensure that the joint is water-tight. Applying plenty of glue to both surfaces and rotating the joint seemed to provide the best join. Glue goes everywhere but can be wiped off provided you move quickly – but the priority should be to get a good joint.

3. Leaks from these pipes happen. The ball valves, equipment joints and couplings are all easily and usually well-sealed. The pipework leaks are usually small drips – annoying, but they do not lose a lot of water.

4. If you leave sufficient space between any two joints you can replace a leaking joint and fit a coupling if necessary, but this extra space does make your pump room much larger.

5. Coating the leaking joint with Griffin glue doesn't work unless you can overlay the joint with further plastic to make a joint on top of a joint.

6. 'Araldite' (a resin glue) **does** work. When mixed this produces a white paste. It is white because it is full of air bubbles. Heating (using a hairdryer) will remove those and strengthen the joint. You must leave 24 hours for the resin to solidify before putting the pipe under pressure. Since Araldite will take pressure it can be successful - particularly at the low pressure end of the pipework (i.e. after the heater and filter).

Appendix 4: Idealised testing regime

- Is the pool Clear and Clean? → Vacuum and Clean
- Clean and recalibrate the pH and ORP meters. Store them in the correct solution.
- Is TDS < 500 ppm?   Is pH 7.4 +/- 0.2?   Is temperature at 29° C?
- Is Hardness = 240 ppm and Alkalinity = 120 ppm?
  Use ORENDA app to calculate additions to take the LSI close to zero
- Backwash or drain and refill | Adjust pH to 7.4 | Check ASHP

pH at 7.4 / Chlorine = 0 ppm / ORP < 400 mV
→ Needs chlorine to kill the bugs. 100G would be a 'shock' dose. 30 G / 4 days is an effective amount. 0.5 ppm is the theoretical level

pH at 7.4 / Chlorine > 1 ppm / ORP < 400 mV
→ Enough chlorine should be available. ORP is low - Does the meter need cleaning and recalibrating?

Could be that the bi-products of chlorination (bits of algae, bits of bacteria,) or even body butter and stuff, is eating up the chlorine. Use enzymes to remove these. Check ORP and chlorine the next day.

Is there algae in the pool? Use the algaeside to kill it, then, 24 hours later, enzymes to break up the bits left over (this will release phosphates from the algae back into the water). Finally, 24 hours after that, add the phosphate-remover to clear the algae's food source.

Check phosphates < 0.1 ppm and copper < 0.5 ppm (The algaeside is copper based)

pH at 7.4 / Chlorine ~1 ppm / ORP ~ 700 mV → Exactly right!

Appendix 5: Spreadsheet for monitoring the pool chemistry

	Measurements of the Pool Water Chemicals												Chemical Additions & Other Actions						
	Temp	pH	TDS	ORP	Free Cl	Total Cl	Chloram	Hardness	Total Alk	LSI	Copper	Phosph	Nitrate	pH	Chlorine	Total Alk	Hard	Enzymes	Phos	Nitrate
Units / Target	°C		ppm	mV	ppm	ppm	ppm	ppm	ppm		ppm	ppm	ppm	inc/dec Gms	inc/dec Gms	inc/dec Gms	inc/dec Gms	Addition	Removal	Removal
Date & Time	29	7.4	<500	700	1.0	0.5	0.5	240	110	0.00	0.5	0	0							

* Measure in flowing water e.g. inside the skimmer with the pump on, or by waving the water past the meter's probe. Wait for the reading to settle.

Appendix 6: Indicative Prices and Costs in £s.

The main pump room equipment was bought from AGBudget and the contact there, Bill (0208 941 6618), was very helpful in identifying the right items as well as with problems or general queries.

These prices, in £s, should be taken as a guide only. There are multiple equipment manufacturers as well as dealers and eBay sales channels.

The Pool Equipment

Excavation, concrete, brickwork and drains (estimated total spend)	2500
Electrical equipment and installation (estimated total spend)	2000
Pond liner, X-Pool Insulation and underlay	600
Liner & Lock	315
Cover roller and straps	120
Pool Cover	186
Steps (actually dive-steps for the back of a boat)	50
SureSet Flooring	550
Stainless steel and glass Balustrade	450

Pump Room Equipment

3/4HP Pentair Pump and 20" Mega filter	565
SeaMaid lights	400
Certikin Skimmer	120
Jetvag Superfast swimjet	1570
HydroPro Plus Premium 10 Air Source Heat Pump (ASHP)	1650

Blue Lagoon UV- Cu Ioniser 75W	730
15 ball valves & 2 non-return valves	300
90 and 45 degree bends (35), and Tee's (15) (estimated numbers)	100
Pipes (15Mts), simple (10) and O-ring (5) joints (estimated numbers)	100
Certikin vacuum, input and outlet eyeballs (estimated numbers)	100
Vacuuming kit	130

Chemical Measurement Equipment

Hanna pH /ORP/ Temperature meter	270
Hanna Free Chlorine HI-701 Colorimeter	52
Hanna HI-711 Total Chlorine Colorimeter	77
Hanna PRIMO Pocket TDS Tester	55
Hanna HI-3841 Hardness Colourimeter	11
Palintest Total Alkalinity 250 Tablets - AS072 (ebay)	48
Seachem MultiTest Phosphate (ebay)	10

Hanna do provide a range of complete test kits and it is worth talking to their Technical Support team.

Chemicals

Blue Horizons Filter Cleaner	£13/Lt
Gold Horizons Enzyme	£30/Lt
Clear 'N Clean algaecide	£22/Lt

Blue Horizons PhosAway	£26/Lt
Sodium Carbonate (soda ash) – to increase pH - Na_2CO_3	£12/Kg
Sodium Bisulphate (dry acid) – to decrease pH - $NaHSO_4$	£8/Kg
Sodium Bisulphate (dry acid) – to lower Total Alkalinity (TA) - $NaHSO_4$	£8/Kg
Calcium Chloride – to increase Hardness - $CaCl_2$	£17/Kg
Calcium Hypochlorite (without CYA stabiliser) - $Ca(ClO)_2$	£20/Kg
Sodium dichloroisocyanurate ($C_3Cl_2N_3NaO_3$) or trichloroisocyanurate ($C_3Cl_3N_3O_3$) – chlorine that includes CYA	£5/Kg
Lo-Chlor No More Metal	£20/Lt
Sodium Bicarbonate – to raise Total Alkalinity (TA) – $NaHCO_3$	£4/Kg

Appendix 7: Some Useful References and sources of Interesting Articles.

Myron L Co. "Ground-breaking Measurement of Free Chlorine Disinfecting Power in a Handheld Instrument". In the Tech section of their website Myron L Company. You may have to contact them to get a copy of this 2012 White Paper.

Eutech Instruments Pty Ltd . "Excellent advice and guidance". See their technical factsheet on Oxidation-reduction potential

AGBudget.   Very helpful equipment supplier

Hanna Instruments. "Outstanding instrumentation"

Orenda Tech. "Excellent advice and guidance".

Pool Help. "Excellent advice and guidance"

APSP. The association of pool and spa professionals - now the 'Pool and Hot Tub Alliance'

Printed in Great Britain
by Amazon